The Vaccine Controversy

The History, Use, and Safety of Vaccinations

Kurt Link, M.D.

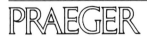

Westport, Connecticut
London

Library of Congress Cataloging-in-Publication Data

Link, Kurt, 1937–
   The vaccine controversy : the history, use, and safety of vaccinations / Kurt
Link.
      p. cm.
   Includes bibliographical references and index.
   ISBN 0-275-98472-9 (alk. paper)
   1. Vaccination.   2. Vaccination—History.   3. Vaccination—
Complications.   4. Vaccines—Health aspects.   5. Vaccines—Safety measures.
   [DNLM: 1. Vaccines—adverse effects.   2. Vaccination—adverse
effects.   3. Vaccination—trends.   4. Vaccines—immunology.]   I. Title.
RA638.L565   2005
614.4'7—dc22   2005003458

British Library Cataloguing in Publication Data is available.

Library of Congress Catalog Card Number: 2005003458
ISBN: 0-275-98472-9

First published in 2005

Praeger Publishers, 88 Post Road West, Westport, CT 06881
An imprint of Greenwood Publishing Group, Inc.
www.praeger.com

Printed in the United States of America

The paper used in this book complies with the
Permanent Paper Standard issued by the National
Information Standards Organization (Z39.48-1984).

10   9   8   7   6   5   4   3   2

To *Gabriella Elizabeth Corbett*
and *Jude Riley Link*

Contents

PART 3: Special Vaccines   127

Introduction

Our hunter-gatherer prehistoric ancestors had hard lives and suffered many injuries, and probably had occasional sporadic illnesses, but they were not subject to infectious plagues and epidemics.

Infectious disease began to appear with the shift to an agrarian society, which included close contact with domestic and other animals. Transmission of infectious agents from animals to man began soon after and continues to this day.[1]

The rise of towns, with its crowding of people together has made possible the transmission of infections from human to human. When the number of cases passes a critical threshold, like kindling erupts into a blaze, an epidemic erupts in the community. If the infection is highly contagious, and if there is travel in and out of the affected community, the epidemic may spread to become a worldwide pandemic. When a disease persists in a population for a long time, the disease is said to be endemic.

The "common source" epidemic is not transmitted from person to person but arises from a common source such as contaminated water.

The number of persons infected and the duration of the epidemic depends on several factors, including the ease of transmission, the incubation period and the proportion of susceptible and immune persons. When the number of immune survivers increases sufficiently, the chain of transmission is broken, and the epidemic stops, even though there are still many susceptible persons. This concept goes by the unfortunate name of herd immunity. The goal of vaccination has been just that: to immunize enough of the population so that transmission can not take place. A new goal is disease eradication, achieved only in the case of smallpox.[2]

The attempt to prevent disease by immunization has a long history. The first well-documented attempts were in seventeenth-century China.

Children were deliberately infected with a mild case of smallpox in the hope of preventing a severe case later. Powdered smallpox scabs or the fluid from a smallpox blister were inserted into the nostril; an alternative method was to have the healthy child wear the underclothes of a sick child. Although the practitioners had no way of knowing it, they were using an attenuated pathogenic live virus vaccine no different in concept from many vaccines used today.

Edward Jenner's vaccine was different. He infected his subjects with cowpox, a mild illness, which resembles smallpox closely enough that immunization of one protects against the other. Jenner's crude experiments (which would not be permitted today on ethical grounds), did stimulate interest in immunization worldwide. The word *vaccinia,* after all, derives from *vacca,* Latin for cow. The early vaccines were developed by an empirical trial and error method (and still are to some extent).

Major advances in vaccine development had to wait for advances in bacteriology and especially virology. Bacteria are easy to grow. Just put some agar in a Petri dish and put it on the window sill—we all did it in high school. Viruses, on the other hand, can only survive in living animal cells, and scientists did not know how to grow them in the lab. In the 1940s and 1950s the problem of growing viruses in the laboratory was finally solved. Chick embryo cells could be cultured and kept alive in a culture of suspended minced kidney in chicken soup; this would support the growth of the virus. The importance of this discovery cannot be overstated: It opened up the golden age of vaccine development. During the following decades the various types of vaccines were developed. The types included live vaccines, killed whole vaccines, purified component vaccines, and anti-toxin vaccines.

At the same time, the immune system was being discovered bit-by-bit. The immune system consists of many components including at least a dozen different kinds of immune cells, a veritable pharmacopea of antibodies, and other chemicals which interact with each other and the cells that produce them. The whole system is coordinated by stimulators, inhibitors and multiple feedback loops all under the ultimate control of the brain. As researchers find out more about how this all works, it should be possible to develop better vaccines.

Success followed upon success. Smallpox, measles, diphtheria, whooping cough, rabies, tetanus, polio—killers all—bit the dust. Life expectancy increased dramatically. Vaccines were the glory of medicine.

Now they are the worry of medicine. Why is it, now that vaccines are safer and more effective than ever before, there is so much trouble? New ideas and methods challenge the old and entrenched. Change is frightening. Many great advances in our civilization are met with opposition. Jenner certainly experienced that, but should the same battle be going on 200 years later? As we shall see, there are many reasons for the current antivaccination activity.

Immunization takes pride of place when it comes to entanglement in religion, philosophy, politics, and the vested interests of doctors, researchers, pharmacists, vaccine manufacturers, the federal and state governments, and malpractice lawyers.

The on-again off-again shortage of flu vaccine in 2004–2005 has caused confusion and alarm. The requirement that the military be vaccinated with anthrax vaccine is tied up in court. The smallpox vaccine fever before the Iraq war has fizzled out. There are plans to produce millions of doses for this nonexistent disease. There are rumors that autism is caused by MMR, or measles, or mercury. There are shortages of several vaccines. Pharmaceutical houses are getting out of the vaccine business because it is not profitable.[3] Experts are predicting the evolution of a new flu strain which will dwarf the horrific pandemics of the past.

Some vaccine troubles arise from their success. As the number of cases decreases, the rate of side effects remains the same. There comes a point when the risk of side effects is greater than the risk of disease. When this happened with smallpox, immunization was discontinued. Polio may soon be in the same category. Thanks to vaccines, the actual illnesses may soon be only memories, but this is likely to decrease vaccination rates.

Some vaccine troubles arise from their failures. I have cataloged extensively the adverse reactions and the disasters that have been the price of progress in immunization therapy. Besides the concern about "usual" adverse reactions like sore arms, fevers, and rashes, there are other issues. Vaccinating babies and children has the effect of shifting upward the age at which individuals may become ill. Mild illnesses of children can be devastating in the adult. This is an issue far from resolved.

I worry that in the future, if children are protected against all childhood ilnesses, they may not get the stimulation needed to develop a mature immune system. A related issue is the creation of highly susceptible populations. Before smallpox was eradicated there were many immune survivors. As we noted, such individuals tend to dampen an epidemic. Now the whole world's population is susceptible; if the smallpox virus returned, we would be immunological pushovers.

This book deals primarily with current disease prevention vaccination practices in the developed nations. It will soon be out of date. Traditional vaccines continue to improve and expand. Purified DNA itself will be the essence of vaccines which will be free of impurities of every kind. New designer vaccines will be created by genetic engineering. Vaccines will be used for treating established infections when prevention has failed.

Infections are rampant in Third World countries. Existing vaccines are not used and the tripod killers—malaria, HIV, and TB—will require new approaches.

Immunologic therapies will be developed against cancer, autoimmune diseases, and other chronic afflictions.

Unfortunately, the new advances will be accompanied by new toxicities; it will take wisdom as well as expertise to maximize the benefit to mankind.

PART 1

Overview

CHAPTER 1

The Immune System and Surviving Infection

Vaccines work, when they do, by having effects on the immune system. The immune system is a complex balance of cells and chemicals that interact to respond to real or imagined threats to our health. The technical immunity literature speaks of more complicated things such as cytokines, leukotrines, interferon alpha, apoptosis, tumor necrosis factor, immunoglobulins, and heavy chains. However, here are some basics that do not take an immunologist to understand.

Ordinarily, when in good health, we make our daily rounds unaware that we do so in an invisible cloud of potentially dangerous microorganisms. Even when no one is sneezing or coughing in the elevator, every breath of air brings viruses and other germs into our lungs. Skin is the rich topsoil for abundant growths of a variety of bacteria, fungi, yeasts, and microscopic parasites. The mouth, even immediately after flossing, brushing, and gargling with an antiseptic mouthwash, is home to the many species that make up the mouth's "normal flora," which, as every emergency room doctor knows, makes a human bite a particularly dangerous variety of animal bite. The colon is home to billions of E. coli bacteria.

We are unaware of all this because the immune system, by contrast, is fully aware, always at work. The moment the immune system weakens or fails, the yeast on skin may cause athlete's foot, the bacteria in an intestine cause diarrhea, the anaerobic bacteria in your mouth cause pyorrhea.

The immune system keeps in check the normal flora; a fungus toenail or halitosis (bad breath) represent only minor lapses. What happens when there is serious damage to the immune system? AIDS is one example. In the early days of the AIDS epidemic, before we had effective treatments, we could only watch as the HIV infection progressed, destroying the person's immune system. Each AIDS sufferer became an unwilling host to all kinds of infections, even ones caused by microorganisms that are ordinarily harmless. Yeasts, protozoa, tuberculosis, and microorganisms in the soil, on food, and in the air infected the brain, lungs, and other organs.

AIDS is not the only common form of immune suppression. Bone marrow transplantation and some cancer chemotherapies temporarily cause severe immune deficiency. Patients undergoing these treatments sometimes need "reverse" isolation to protect them from the bacteria that healthy people carry. Cancer specialists have learned to treat these patients intensely with antibiotics at the first sign of infection (usually fever).

Children born with some kinds of severe immune deficiency could survive, until recent advances in treatment, only by living in a plastic bubble, never to directly touch another human. Even the body's "normal flora" can kill these children. Recent advances in gene therapy, however, hold some hope for a cure.

A less well known role of the immune system is prevention of cancer. As soon as the immune system detects a cancer cell, it attempts to destroy it. This function of the immune system was discovered, in part, when physicians noticed that kidney transplant patients had more cancers than expected. These and other transplant patients are treated with immunosuppressive medications to prevent rejection of the transplant. It became apparent that any prolonged weakness of the immune system, including HIV infection, is associated with an increased cancer rate.

These are some of the results of blunted immune responses. But unusually heightened immune responses also have problematic effects. Consider allergic reactions. The symptoms of hay fever are not due to the ragweed pollen, which is harmless. The symptoms are due to the immune system's delusion that the pollen is out to kill, so it makes an all-out counterattack on the pollen. Part of that attack consists of liberating histamine and other chemicals that cause the sneezing, runny nose, and itchy eyes. Asthma, eczema, and hives are other signs of the immune system gone awry. Although penicillin is harmless (except in massive doses), many of its users have died because of a misguided, hyperreactive immune system, which caused anaphylactic shock.

Autoimmunity is another result of abnormal immune responses. In this case the immune system attacks itself or the tissues of its owner. Some forms of anemia, arthritis, kidney disease, and endocrine diseases such as thyroid disease, diabetes, or Addison's disease may result.

So let us look at the components of the immune system and how they work. The immune responses are incredibly complicated, having evolved during the millions of years in which humans have had to learn how to ward off pathogenic bacteria, viruses, and parasites.

INNATE IMMUNITY

We all have certain innate defenses against invasion by microbes and poisons. These defenses are innate in the sense that they are present in everyone and are not directed against any particular infections or toxins. They react to all "foreigners" the same, making no distinctions. We will see later how innate immunity differs from *acquired immunity*.

The first goal of innate immunity is to prevent poisons or microbes from entering the body. The skin is, of course, our great protector. When intact, it is a powerful mechanical defense. However, when it is damaged, as for example, by a scratch, a puncture, or a burn, it can allow bacteria such as "staph" to enter the body and bloodstream, causing the some-times-fatal "blood poisoning" of the pre-antibiotic days. (The emergence of bacteria resistant to penicillin and other antibiotics threatens to bring back those bad old days.) The skin is also a chemical barrier, producing lactic acid and other chemicals that inhibit or destroy some bacteria.

Invasion of the body may occur by not only penetration of the skin but also by penetration of the lining of the eyelids, mouth, and internal organs, including the intestinal, respiratory, and genital and urinary tracts. These linings, or mucous membranes, are the critical boundaries between the inside and the outside of the body. They are in constant contact with myriad potentially infectious agents in the air, food, and the stool in the intestines.

Many microbes, for example, cause infection by penetrating the lung. These invaders must overcome the respiratory tract's mechanical defenses, which include a vigorous cough reflex, which expels foreign material. Additional protection comes from the microscopic hairlike cilia in the bronchial tubes. They sweep out foreign matter trapped in the mucus secreted by special cells.

Enzymes known as lysozymes, present in tears and saliva, protect the eyes and mouth. These enzymes can kill some bacteria and parasites, preventing disease and incidentally decreasing the likelihood of transmitting infection by saliva.

The stomach is protected by the production of hydrochloric acid, which kills most bacteria (but not the Helicobacter pylori recently discovered to be the cause of many stomach and duodenal ulcers).

These common innate immune mechanisms are our fortress. Unfortunately, sometimes the fortress is breached and infectious agents make their way inside. Once inside the body, these agents face two kinds of protective forces: cells and chemicals.

One type of cell is the *natural killer* cell, usually called NK cell. This remarkable cell patrols all the tissues of the body and has the ability to detect subtle changes on the surface of cells that have become cancerous or in which bacteria or viruses are hiding. The NK cells kill the infected cell or bacteria by attaching to them and secreting a chemical that makes holes in their outer membrane; water rushes in, the cell swells and finally bursts.

Alternatively, the NK cell injects chemicals into the sick cell, inducing cell suicide by activating the *death domain* that exists in most cells in the human body. Activation of the death domain triggers a chemical chain reaction that causes the cell to literally fall apart. This cell suicide, called *apoptosis*, can be switched on in various ways and is one way the body controls the growth and longevity of many cells.

In addition to the NK, white blood cells join the attack. Some release chemicals into the blood, alerting distant cells to rush to the breach. These compounds also increase the flow of blood to the infected organ and cause the capillary cells to loosen their connection with each other so that more white blood cells can escape.

Other white cells, *phagocytes*, swallow the bacteria and destroy them by walling them off in internal sacs filled with toxic superoxide ions, hydrogen peroxide, and killing enzymes. This process occurs in minutes and is associated with a tremendous burst of energy. There is an illness known as *chronic granulomatous disease* in which the phagocytes cannot manufacture the superoxide ions. The affected persons are subjected to a lifetime of recurrent sinus, bronchial, and other infections.

The protective effect of the white cells is dramatized by the plight of patients who have too few, because of chemotherapy, leukemia, or other conditions. These patients must be protected (by reverse isolation) from everyday, ordinarily harmless germs, which can, in this case, cause fatal infections.

The chemical defenses of innate immunity include compounds that attach to the surface of bacteria, making them sticky and rough and so easier for the phagocytes to ingest.

Other chemical reactions may come into play. Some bacteria, to their regret, initiate a cascade of approximately twenty proteins, the *complement system,* which ultimately produces chemicals known as the *membrane attack complex* (MAC). The MAC splits, weakens, and causes the cell membrane to become leaky, finally killing the cell.

These are the chief elements of innate immunity: the barriers of skin and mucous membranes, the NK and other white blood cells, complement and other protective chemical compounds. The absence or failure of any one of these elements results in vulnerability to infections.

ACQUIRED IMMUNITY

We have reviewed innate immunity—the immunologic armor issued at birth to all healthy people. Anther type of immunity is *acquired immunity*. The Greek historian Thucydides noted that when the plague was raging in Athens in the fifth century B.C., nursing care was provided by dedicated and compassionate individuals who had the plague and survived, for it was known that no one caught the plague twice. Thucydides did not know why this was true; today we have some clues. These individuals had developed immunity that is acquired during the course of an infection and prevents reinfection with the same organism. This is also the kind of immunity acquired after successful vaccination, so an understanding of how it works will help us understand why vaccines work or don't work.

There are four basic concepts that we can define and discuss: *immune specificity; immune memory; cellular immunity; and humoral immunity.*

Immune specificity means that the immune response is targeted to a specific infection. You may be immune to smallpox, but not chicken pox; you may be immune to regular measles but not German measles, and so on. This specificity means that the immune response is more like a rifle than a blunderbuss and so will not hit the wrong target. But there is a downside to this specificity. Some viruses have learned to escape our immune defense by changing their surface in such a way that the immune cells cannot recognize them. So, if you are infected with the Hong Kong flu and acquire immunity to it, the next year the flu virus comes back changed slightly to, say, the avian flu. Your immune system fails to detect the similarity and you get the flu again. This is why the flu vaccine must be taken every year. It is not because the vaccine has worn off; it is because each flu season there is a new variety of the virus, and so a new vaccine is needed.

In the case of the common cold, there are over one hundred varieties of virus that can cause cold symptoms, so although it appears that colds recur, in reality most of the time the "recurrence" is due to an infection with a different virus.

Some bacteria present a different problem. They do not keep changing, but they do have multiple varieties. The pneumococcus, which causes many cases of bacterial pneumonia, exists in eighty-four different types. Immunity against one does not protect against the others. To be completely effective in such a case, a vaccine would have to stimulate immunity to all the types, a practical impossibility. Fortunately, it is not necessary to protect against all eighty-four types because over 85 percent of infections (including the most virulent types) are cause by twenty-three of the types.

Modern pneumococcal vaccines are designed to stimulate immunity to these twenty-three types.

Immune specificity, as we shall see, comes about because certain cells of the immune system recognize and react to only one type of bacteria or other pathogen.

The second concept is immune memory. The first time you have any specific infection, it takes 6–12 days for the immune system to react effectively. The next time you meet the same agent, the response is much faster and stronger because the immune system remembers the first exposure and is prepared. After the first exposure, the immune memory may be imperfect and may in time "forget." After the second exposure, the memory is imprinted more intensely and the immune system may never forget again. This is an important concept because vaccines may produce a weaker immune response and weaker memory than natural infection. Booster shots are often used to overcome this problem. The immune memory may also be impaired if an infection is treated with antibiotics before the full immune response has developed. In that case, the treatment, although effective, leaves you susceptible to reinfection.

The third concept is cellular immunity, mediated by the billions of *lymphocytes* in the blood and tissues throughout the body. These cells recognize the foreign or "nonself." This "recognition" involves structures *(receptors)* on the surface of the lymphocyte that connect with complementary structures *(antigens)* on the surface of the infectious or toxic agent. The connection has been likened to the fit between a lock and key. The controversy centers on how the lymphocyte acquires the necessary receptors. The most widely accepted theory is that there are many millions of different lymphocytes, each with a preformed, unique structure. There are so many of these that at least one lymphocyte is likely to have the receptor to fit the antigen of any infectious agent on earth. Once stimulated by the appropriate antigen, the lymphocyte begins to multiply rapidly, so stimulation of even one lymphocyte may be sufficient to elicit a strong reaction.

Some of the lymphocytes, *T cells,* so named because they mature in the thymus gland in the neck, participate in the immune response by secreting various substances when they encounter an infectious agent or foreign material. These substances marshal additional help to assist phagocytes in ingesting and killing bacteria, stimulate the natural killer cells, and stimulate antibody production. These cells are the *T helper* cells that are targeted by the HIV virus. Other T cells, *T regulatory* cells, control and regulate the overall immune response; they can dampen or even turn off a response that is excessive. The properly regulated response depends on the interaction of these two systems.

Other T cells transform into *cytotoxic lymphocytes,* much like the natural killer cells, but these, unlike the natural killer cells, become active only when they contact an agent to which they have been sensitized. Like the natural killer cells, the cytotoxic lymphocytes attach themselves to bacteria or cells containing bacteria or viruses and destroy them with membrane-dissolving chemicals.

Another type of lymphocyte, arising from the bone marrow, is the *B lymphocyte,* or *B cell.* Some of these cells, when stimulated by a foreign antigen, and with the help of T helper cells, become *plasma cells* that produce the antibodies that are crucial to the recovery from and the prevention of many common infections. When actively fighting an infection, plasma cells can secrete thousands of antibody molecules per second for hours at a time.

Other B cells become memory cells. They leave the fray for the safety of the lymph nodes, where they reside indefinitely. They carry the memory of past infections and are prepared to activate and proliferate at a moment's notice if the enemy reappears.

The final concept is humoral immunity. This refers to the antibodies circulating in the blood. Antibodies cling to and coat the infectious agent, killing it in the process, either making it easier for phagocytes to ingest or simply preventing it from attacking the host's cells. Antibodies to specific infectious agents begin to appear several days after the infection starts.

Their appearance usually heralds the beginning of recovery. Antibodies also appear after successful immunization. In fact, measuring the antibody level is the best way to tell if a vaccination has been successful.

There are several types of antibodies: Some show up early in infection, some later; some are associated with parasitic infections, others with allergic reactions. One type, known as immunoglobulin (antibody) A is of particular interest with regard to vaccines. Immunoglobulin A is present mainly on the lining of the respiratory and intestinal tracts, where it is the first line of defense against infectious agents inhaled or swallowed. This defense is bypassed by vaccines that are injected, and so in this regard the response to a vaccine is different from natural infection.

The immune response is weaker at the beginning and at the end of our natural life span. The newborn has an immature immune system that does not become fully functional until it is exposed to viruses and bacteria; lack of such exposure may distort the immune responses. Our discussion of vaccines later in the book will discuss this point further. On the other hand, as we get older, our immune system, like many other bodily functions, loses some of its vigor.

The immune response is a highly complex interaction of innate immunity and acquired immunity, involving many different blood cells, chemicals, and antibodies. It is this complexity that gives us the power and flexibility needed to ward off the infectious agents that surround us.

CHAPTER 2

Vaccine History and Types

Here we will take a generic look at immunization. Specific vaccines will be used to illustrate certain points, but we will defer detailed descriptions of the common vaccines until later chapters.

The history of vaccines always starts with the smallpox story. Smallpox, caused by a virus, is an ancient ailment. In its severe form the affliction starts with high fever. Three or four days later blisters and pus sores begin to appear, first on the palms and feet, then moving to the center of the body, and finally spreading all over, including the head and face. Headache, backache, abdominal pain, vomiting, confusion, and coma precede a painful death. Some epidemics have mortality rates above 80 percent; others are much less virulent. Survivors carry the scars and deformity for life.

Smallpox is the infection that prompted the first attempt to induce protective immunity. More than one thousand years ago, Chinese healers practiced what is now called "variolation." The idea was to deliberately cause a mild case of the disease to protect the individual from contracting the natural, severe disease. The method used by these early practitioners was to blow some dried matter from a pox pustule into the nostrils of the recipient, hoping to induce an uncomplicated form of smallpox.

In the early eighteenth century, Lady Mary Wortley Montague, wife of the now forgotten Turkish ambassador, learned of "smallpox parties," which she described in a letter to a friend back home in England: "The smallpox, so fatal and general among us, here is entirely harmless by the invention of engrafting [variolation]. There is a set of old women who make it their business to perform the operation every autumn in the month of September when the great heat is abated....They make parties for the purpose...the old woman comes with a nutshell full of the matter of the best sort of smallpox, and asks what veins you please have open'd.

She immediately rips open . . . and puts into the vein as much [smallpox] matter as can lie upon the head of her needle."[1]

Lady Mary was so enthusiastic about this procedure that she brought it to Britain, where she had her five-year-old son inoculated. During the ensuing thirty years, some four hundred thousand persons were variolated, and the number of smallpox cases decreased markedly. Among the elite, variolation developed into an elaborate, costly, irrational, ritualized procedure in which children were confined to so-called hospitals for weeks on end for bleeding, purging, starving, and purifying before the inoculation, and then confined until any sores or illness resolved. Edward Jenner was one of the many children subjected to this procedure. Jenner, years later a country doctor in England, is credited with developing the first vaccine, made from a related cowpox, that made people resistant to smallpox.

In time the popularity of variolation diminished, partly because of the 1 percent to 3 percent death rate associated with the occasional severe reactions (which could spread smallpox to others) and partly because of the greater safety and efficacy of Jenner's cowpox vaccine. Ultimately variolation actually became a felony.

Variolation was the first successful attempt to deliberately induce immunity to an infection. The material used, however, was the smallpox virus itself, unlike vaccines, which do not use live native viruses or bacteria. The beginning of modern vaccination was Jenner's demonstration that deliberately infecting a person with cowpox, which causes a mild localized infection, would protect against smallpox infection. The word vaccine incidentally comes from the Latin word for cow (vacca), a reminder that the first true vaccine was the cowpox virus. We will explore this story in greater detail later.

TYPES OF VACCINES

There are more than thirty vaccines licensed in the United States. There are several types, including live vaccine or live bacteria; killed whole virus or killed whole bacteria; purified components (subunits) of virus or bacteria; and toxoids. All have unique advantages and disadvantages. Let us consider each in turn.

VIRUS VACCINES

In the pre–World War II decades of the twentieth century, viruses were grown by infecting live animals, most often ferrets and mice. Vaccines were prepared from the tissues of these animals, including mouse brain and lung. Not surprisingly, many of these early vaccines were dangerous or ineffective, or both dangerous and ineffective at the same time. Modern virus vaccines are made from viruses grown in the laboratory. Since viruses live and grow only in living cells, these vaccines could be developed only in the fifties, after the discovery of tissue culture.

While working in the zoology laboratories of Yale in the 1930s, Ross Granville Harrison developed a method of lining a glass or plastic surface with a single layer of living animal cells. Another method was to use enzymes to break tiny pieces of animal tissues into single cells and suspend them in a nourishing biologic medium such as lymph, blood plasma, serum, or tissue juices. Once animal cells could be grown in tissue culture, it became possible to grow viruses in the laboratory. Viruses for vaccines are commonly grown in cells from monkey kidney, chick embryo, and human fetus. Cells from an embryo or fetus are easier to maintain in culture than are fully matured and differentiated cells.

One of the problems with animal cell tissue culture is the potential presence of contamination by undetected animal viruses. Indeed, in the early days of polio vaccine development such a contamination did occur, and millions of individuals were and still are infected with the SV monkey virus. This infection has long been considered harmless, but recently there has been suspicion that after ten or more years there may be an increase in brain cancers. This will be discussed later in the book.

LIVE VIRUS VACCINES

Live virus vaccines contain a harmless, attenuated strain of the wild, disease-causing virus. The attenuated virus resembles the wild virus so closely that antibodies against the vaccine virus will cross-protect against the wild virus.

The wild virus may be attenuated by various manipulations in the laboratory, such as repeatedly diluting and regrowing the culture or by passing the virus through different species of animal cells that are not the virus's natural host Another way to attenuate the wild virus is to grow it in unnatural conditions such as high or very low temperatures. A cold-adapted attenuated flu virus has been used as a vaccine in Russia.

Instead of using attenuated viruses, animal viruses similar to human disease viruses have been used as vaccines. The first vaccine in history was the use of cowpox to immunize against smallpox. No other similar success has been achieved, although viruses similar to the diarrhea-causing human rotavirus have been isolated from rhesus monkeys and cows and used in experimental vaccines. The monkey virus caused fever and diarrhea, and the cow virus raised antibodies in only 75 percent of children and was never licensed.[2]

In some ways, live virus vaccines are the best. Even one dose triggers a very strong and long-lasting (even lifelong) immunity similar to natural infection. (Live polio vaccine is an exception; multiple doses are required to induce immunity to all three types of poliovirus.) Oral live viral vaccines, like natural infection, stimulate the production of IgA antibodies on the mucosal surfaces of the mouth, throat, lungs, intestinal tract, and urinary system, protecting the body from penetration by infectious agents.

One problem with live vaccines is that children less than one year of age may have a weak or absent response because the mother's antibodies may persist in the infant, preventing the vaccine from "taking."

There are some serious downsides to live vaccines. The harmless vaccine may not be so harmless to individuals who have a depressed immune system as occurs in HIV infection, some cancers, chemotherapy patients, or patients taking cortisone-like medication. In those cases the vaccine virus may cause serious, even fatal, infections. Live vaccines should not be given to such persons.

Sometimes the "harmless" virus may cause serious infection even in apparently healthy individuals, as happens regularly, but rarely after oral polio vaccination. In recent years the live vaccine has caused all the cases of paralytic polio in the U.S. There is the additional worry that the vaccine virus may revert to the "wild" natural invasive form. This may have occurred in the case of the Urabe strain of the mumps vaccine, which caused cases of meningitis before its withdrawal. On the other hand, if too attenuated, the vaccine may fail to protect the body from natural infection. This has been the case with a different mumps vaccine, the Rubini strain.[3]

Another feature of live vaccines is that they may spread from a recently vaccinated person to close contacts. This can be a good feature in that it vaccinates the contact, but it can be not so good if the contact is immunosuppressed. Smallpox vaccine virus can spread to contacts. Rubella vaccine virus (German measles) has been transmitted via breast milk and may possibly be spread by coughing or sneezing. Measles and mumps live vaccines are not known to spread to contacts. Live vaccines should not be given to individuals who have household or other close contacts with people who have impaired immunity.

Some common live virus vaccines are measles, rubella (German measles), mumps, oral polio, and chicken pox.

LIVE BACTERIAL VACCINES

In the case of bacteria, which are more complex microbes than are viruses, scientists have had less success in developing attenuated harmless strains that can be used as vaccines.

The first live bacterial vaccine was the vaccine against tuberculosis. The BCG tuberculosis vaccine is a strain of the bacterium that causes cow tuberculosis, Mycobacterium bovis, which was attenuated by 231 passages through various culture mediums. Current stocks of BCG are direct descendants of the original strain isolated in the early twentieth century. The vaccine became available for human use in 1927. Researchers have made many attempts to develop other live bacterial vaccines, but most strains have proved too toxic or virulent or else excessively attenuated so that they were ineffective.

Like live oral viral vaccines, live oral bacterial vaccines elicit a strong immune response in the intestinal tract, and the immunity tends to be long-lasting. There are live oral bacterial vaccines for typhoid fever and cholera (licensed abroad but not in the USA).

KILLED WHOLE VACCINES

The active ingredient in this kind of vaccine is the whole, killed organism, which has a variety of surface and internal structures that are strong stimulants of the immune system. This makes for an effective vaccine but also increases the possibility of an allergic reaction. The microbe is killed (often referred to as inactivated) by heat, phenol, formalin, or thimerosal. Since the microbe is killed, this kind of vaccine cannot cause an infection.

Unlike natural infection or some live vaccines, killed vaccines require multiple doses initially to induce immunity and booster doses later to maintain immunity. Another drawback is that killed vaccines do not stimulate the mucosal surface antibodies the way a live vaccine or natural infection does. As a result, an individual may acquire a nose or throat infection (such as pertussis, the cause of whooping cough) that does not cause illness because the vaccine-induced immunity prevents the microbe from invading the body. However, persons with this kind of infection without symptoms may be carriers and spread the infection to susceptible individuals.

Anthrax, cholera, Japanese encephalitis, pertussis (whooping cough), plague, rabies, polio (inactivated type), and typhoid vaccines are examples of killed whole vaccines.

PURIFIED VACCINES

These vaccines, sometimes referred to as subunit vaccines, consist of relatively pure chemical components of a microbe. Infectious agents have chemicals on their surface, some of which stimulate antibodies. In the case of bacteria, these are polysaccharides, a form of complex sugars. Viruses on the other hand are usually coated with proteins. In both cases the vaccine is made by purifying these components by straightforward laboratory methods such as filtering, heating, and extracting with various solvents.

A newer method of producing subunit vaccines is to use recombinant technology, a form of genetic engineering. The hepatitis B vaccine is this type. The hepatitis B virus (HBV) has a gene that produces a chemical known as surface antigen. This gene is inserted into yeast cells, which become, in a sense, part hepatitis virus. These recombinant yeasts are "tricked" into manufacturing the hepatitis B surface antigen, which is harvested to produce the vaccine. Yeast cells are easy to grow in the laboratory and make possible the production of large amounts of a very pure vaccine.

An even more advanced type of subunit vaccine, still in the experimental phase, is to insert the genetic material (DNA) in the cells of the person receiving the vaccine, so that the person's own cells produce the vaccine.

Like killed vaccines, these cannot cause infection because they are only a piece of the microbe. These purified vaccines are less likely to have side effects than whole virus vaccines. Their disadvantage is that they stimulate a relatively constricted immune response and may require multiple doses and boosters in order to maintain immunity.

Vaccines against pneumococcal pneumonia, hepatitis B, and hemophilus influenza are in this "purified" category.

TOXOIDS

So far, we have been considering vaccines that stimulate the production of antibodies against an infectious agent. Toxoids on the other hand produce antibodies against toxins secreted by certain bacteria, but not the organism itself.

The tetanus bacterium, for example, produces its often-lethal effect by manufacturing a powerful toxin that causes the dreaded lockjaw. To make the toxoid vaccine, the microbe is grown in huge vats. The toxin it produces is extracted by filtration and other laboratory manipulations. Once the pure toxin has been prepared, it is inactivated by incubating with formalin, producing the toxoid. When injected, the toxoid is nontoxic but stimulates antibodies that will combine with and so neutralize any subsequent exposure to the toxin. Infection with the tetanus germ may still occur, but it is rendered harmless. Common toxoid vaccines include diphtheria and tetanus.

PASSIVE IMMUNITY

We have been considering immunizations that stimulate the body to produce antibodies; this is an active process referred to (no surprise) as active immunity. Passive immunity on the other hand is produced by administering antibodies or antitoxins extracted from the serum of a person (or horse in some cases) who is already immune through natural exposure or immunization. These antibodies will be protective as long as they last in the recipient's body.

Immune human serum globulin (IHSG, "gamma globulin") is the most frequently used antibody preparation. To make sure that there are a maximum number of antibody types present, each lot contains serum from as many as a thousand donors. The problem with this is that the recipient has a thousand chances of receiving antibodies from an infected or contaminated donor. Fortunately, modern methods are able, as far as we know, to eliminate or exclude any viruses or other impurities.

In addition to HSIG, there are special gamma globulin preparations used for specific infections, such as hepatitis, tetanus, and chicken pox. These antibodies are protective as long as they last, which is only days or, at most, weeks.

Antitoxins are another type of antibody. Antitoxins are directed against the toxins produced by bacteria such as diphtheria and tetanus or produced by snakes and spiders. These often lifesaving antitoxins are used primarily to treat persons already exposed to the poison rather than to prevent infection from occurring. To this day antitoxins against diphtheria, botulism, and spider and snake venoms are derived from the serum of horses that have been hypervaccinated. Horse serum, of course, frequently causes adverse reactions, including serum sickness. Diphtheria antitoxin is no longer manufactured or licensed in the USA, but the CCD (Center for Communicable Diseases) has a supply of a French preparation to use in case of an emergency. Until the 1960s, tetanus antitoxin was also derived from horses, but now there is a human-derived preparation.

Passive immunization is often used when there is not enough time to wait for a response from an active vaccine. It is used to protect a susceptible, unimmunized individual just before an anticipated exposure, such as contact with an infected household member, or as soon as possible after an unexpected exposure, such as a hypodermic needle stick or other injury. Active immunization is sometimes begun at the same time. The chief advantage of passive immunity is that it begins to work at once, in contrast to active immunity, which is not protective until the body has had enough time to produce antibodies.

Passive immunization is used to protect against infections caused by the agents of tetanus, diphtheria, rabies, measles, hepatitis A and B, chicken pox, and shingles as well as the noninfection-related toxins of the pit viper snake and black widow spider bites, and botulism.

There is another, natural, form of passive immunity: maternal immunology protection of the newborn and infant. Before birth, the mother's antibodies enter the fetus's bloodstream. At birth, the baby has a complement of the mother's antibodies, which just happen to be directed against the infections prevalent in that environment. The mother may have antibodies due to natural infection or due to immunization, but in either case they are transmitted to the fetus and provide protection during the precarious first six months of life. Immunizing the mother during pregnancy will result in higher antibody levels in the newborn, but vaccinating pregnant women for this purpose is probably not a good or acceptable idea.

Breast-feeding provides more passive immune protection. Human milk is rich in maternal antibodies, especially the kind that are present in the intestinal and respiratory tracts. The adult cannot absorb ingested antibodies, but the infant intestine has modifications that allow the large antibody molecules to pass into the baby's body. Human milk also contains lactoferrin, which functions like a natural broad-spectrum antibiotic. There are other substances, including cytokines and growth factors, that may stimulate and mature the infant's immune system. This may be why breast-fed infants show some protective effect for several years after breast-feeding has been discontinued.[4] Breast-fed children may respond better to vaccines and generally be more resistant to infections. On the other hand, the presence of maternal antibodies has to be taken into account when scheduling vaccinations, since live vaccines may be neutralized by antibodies.

Maternal passive immunity protects infants against cholera, infectious diarrhea, and infections of the respiratory tract, the middle ear, and urine, as well as sepsis (blood poisoning) and colitis.

VACCINE COMPONENTS

The active vaccine, which we have just reviewed, is only one component of the finished vaccine product. Other components are a fluid or other medium to carry the vaccine, preservatives, and adjuvants to boost the immune response. These components have important effects on the potency and toxicity of the vaccines. The same vaccine made by different manufacturers may not be the same at all because of differences in these other components. Indeed, different batches by the same manufacturer may differ as the manufacturing process is changed over time for one or another reason.

Suspending Fluid

The active vaccine is usually suspended in sterile water or saline, but some vaccines are suspended in fluids that contain calf serum, chicken egg protein, or gelatin, which is derived from pig. Each one of these can cause allergic reactions, usually mild but occasionally life-threatening (anaphylaxis). Although current measles and mumps vaccines are derived from chick egg tissue cultures, they contain very little egg protein and rarely cause reactions, even in children who are allergic to eggs. Influenza vaccine on the other hand has been associated with severe egg-allergic reactions. It is possible to skin test to see if there is an allergy to a vaccine, and if the test is positive, an attempt can be made to desensitize the individual by starting with a very dilute vaccine and gradually increasing the dose at five to twenty-minute intervals, but this is a dangerous procedure in which the risk ordinarily far outweighs the benefit.

Preservatives

Preservatives are present in almost all vaccines. They prevent contamination of the vaccine by bacteria and other pathogens. Contamination is most common in multidose vials, which are entered by hypodermic needle repeatedly. Streptococcal ("strep") infections have been caused by the administration of DPT vaccine taken from contaminated multidose vials.[5] Single-dose vials or factory prefilled syringes present less of a risk but are more expensive.

One of the most commonly used preservatives is thimerosal. Thimerosal is a mercury-containing compound with high antibacterial activity. It has been used in vaccines since the 1930s, in millions of doses, without any known toxicity. However, this benign history is not entirely reassuring today.

For one thing, in recent years the number of immunizations, and the accompanying dose of thimerosal, has increased many times over; present recommendations call for at least sixteen injections in the first two years of life. A second factor is the survival of ever smaller premature babies. A fragile newborn weighing five pounds is much less resilient than a robust eight-pounder. The less mature the still developing brain is, the more vulnerable it is to toxins and stress.

The issue of thimerosal toxicity became a hot topic when, in June 1999, the FDA (Food and Drug Administration) revealed that small infants who receive multiple doses of thimerosal-containing vaccines could be exposed to amounts of mercury that exceed some federal guidelines. There are four "official" guidelines: those of the Environmental Protection Agency (EPA), the World Health Organization (WHO), the Food and Drug Administration (FDA), and the Agency for Toxic Substances Disease Registry. Each cites a different value. However, even if the guidelines were not exceeded, there would still be cause for concern because the guidelines are based on poor evidence that has little relevance to infant immunization.

The guidelines refer to methylmercury, but the breakdown product of thimerosal is ethylmercury, which may have a different toxicity.

Epidemics of gross mercury poisoning have taught us much of what we know about mercury toxicity. The Minamata, Japan, epidemic of industrial waste mercury poisoning in the fifties and the epidemic in Iraq in 1971 when farmers ate seeds treated with mercury caused neurological damage, intestinal hemorrhage, and kidney failure.

Other information about mercury toxicity is derived from studies of adults who have had long-term exposure to low levels of mercury by way of eating mercury-contaminated fish.

These may not be good models for evaluating intermittent injections of thimerosal in an infant. More pertinent are the studies[6] of Faeroe Island children. The Faeroese consume much fish and pilot whale blubber and so are exposed to more than usual amounts of mercury. Grandjean estimated prenatal exposure by measuring the mercury content of the mothers' hair. High levels of prenatal exposure result in retardation, palsy, and congenital deformities. However, even children exposed to low, supposedly safe levels of mercury showed, by age seven, subtle defects in brain function, especially in the domains of motor dexterity, language, and memory.

The most controversial clinical issue has been the thimerosal-containing hepatitis B vaccine. The CDC, Public Health Service, and the American Board of Pediatrics had recommended giving the vaccine at birth. The need for this is in itself controversial, but when the mercury issue became known, the recommendation was changed to allow a delay for six months, except in certain high-risk situations.

Partly because of public concern, a thimerosal-free hepatitis B vaccine has been developed and licensed since August 1999, making this issue moot in the USA. However, some vaccines, including some widely used ones (especially in the poorer nations), still contain thimerosal. Thimerosal-containing vaccines used in the U.S. include some DPT, Hemophilus influenza, flu, meningococcal, pneumococcus, and rabies vaccines.

In spite of all the concern, we must remember that there has not been a single case of proven mercury toxicity from vaccines, and that these vaccines save lives. The obvious solution to the problem is the development of thimerosal-free vaccines. The CDC, Public Health Service, and American Board of Pediatrics have called upon the FDA and the pharmaceutical industry to develop, test, and approve thimerosal-free vaccines.

So far we have been considering mercury poisoning, to which anyone is susceptible if exposed to a high enough dose. Allergic reactions also occur. These are due to antithimerosal antibodies and happen only to persons allergic to thimerosal. As is the case in most allergic reactions, these are unpredictable, and the severity of the reaction bears little relation to the dose; a tiny dose can cause a major reaction.

Thimerosal is not the only preservative used in vaccines. Such antibiotics as streptomycin, neomycin, and polymyxin B are in polio and other vaccines. These are toxic drugs but are present in vaccines in such small trace amounts that they are harmless as drugs, but may not be harmless as allergens. An individual allergic to the antibiotic may have an allergic reaction, which is usually a minor rash appearing 48 to 96 hours after administration of the vaccine. Penicillin and its derivatives are not present in any vaccine licensed in the United States.

Adjuvants

An adjuvant (Latin, *adjuvare*: to help) is any substance that intensifies the immune response to another substance, such as a vaccine. In the absence of an adjuvant, some vaccines do not work, especially subunit, purified, highly specific ones. Live vaccines do not require an adjuvant for full efficacy.

In 1912, for reasons unknown, a French scientist, Gaston Ramon, mixed tapioca with an inactivated tetanus toxin and found, in his animal experiments, that this combination was a more powerful immunostimulant than either component alone. Even bread crumbs had the same effect.[7]

In 1937, Jules Freund, working in New York City's Public Health Institute, noted that sometimes animals infected with tuberculosis had an unusually intense reaction to vaccines. Based on this canny observation, Freund developed an adjuvant containing mineral oil, industrial emulsifiers, and killed, dried tuberculosis culture. It was a strange mix, but so effective that "Freund's adjuvant" is still used in laboratories today.

Later, workers found many unrelated substances that are potential adjuvants. Unfortunately, most of these cause an unregulated release of toxic substances associated with inflammation and so are not clinically useful.

Different adjuvants work in different ways, and most work in more than one way, but all bring the immune system in closer contact with the active vaccine components. The adjuvant can act as a depot, slowly releasing and prolonging the effect of the vaccine. Some adjuvants transform vaccines into tiny particles, which are taken up and ingested by specialized immune cells. Ultimately the adjuvant stimulates these antibody-producing cells that start the long series of chain reactions that finally result in new antibodies and/or activated immune cells. Some adjuvants selectively stimulate immune cells in the respiratory or digestive system.

Adjuvants may allow use of lower doses of vaccines, decreasing both cost and toxicity. Although there are many experimental adjuvants, there is at present only one licensed adjuvant: alum, which is a mixture of aluminum hydroxide and aluminum phosphate. It has been used since the 1940s, but we still do not know the details of how it works. Inflammation may occur at the site of injection, but serious toxicity is rare indeed; literally billions of doses have been safely administered.[8]

Researchers are optimistic: The development of better adjuvants will expand the world of clinical immunology to include the untouchable infections caused by bacteria, viruses, and even protozoa such as malaria. Cancer, autoimmune diseases, and other chronic ailments may also respond to the enhanced immunotherapy.

The hazards of vaccination are real. So are the benefits. In the next chapter we will look at these issues more closely.

CHAPTER 3

Disasters and Near Misses

We can consider a small sample of some dramatic and well-documented disasters and near misses involving vaccines. Many more are recorded; others never saw official documentation. The purpose here is not to disparage vaccinations or to provide ammunition to the militant antivaccinationists. Vaccines have done far more good than harm, but an intelligent appraisal is not possible if mishaps are ignored.

MARBLEHEAD, MASSACHUSETTS, 1800

In July 1800, Jenner (see chapter 5) sent a sample of smallpox vaccine to Benjamin Waterhouse in Marblehead Massachusetts. The community was smallpox free, but Waterhouse initiated a vaccination program. At first all went well, but as the summer wore on, more and more severe reactions occurred. By October a frank smallpox epidemic gripped the town and killed sixty-eight of its residents. In retrospect, it appears that the vaccine that Jenner gave to Waterhouse contained an attenuated smallpox virus that reverted to full virulence.

BREMEN, GERMANY, 1893

During a smallpox vaccination campaign in 1893 in the port of Bremen, 1,289 shipyard workers were vaccinated. Apparently the same serum was passed from one patient's pustules to the next patient. Within eight months, 191 of the men developed hepatitis with jaundice. Dr. Lurman, director of the campaign, correctly concluded that the men had experienced a form of hepatitis transferable by human lymph fluid. This initial observation was the beginning of our understanding that some chronic diseases can be transferred by the blood of an infected individual. This led to understanding diseases of blood-borne pathogens, vital in today's medical practice. It was a startling and important discovery.

DALLAS, TEXAS, 1919

Some of the worst disasters have been caused by early diphtheria vaccines. Known as TAM, they were a mixture of diphtheria toxin mixed with antitoxin (toxin-antitoxin mixture). The theory was that the toxin would stimulate antibodies but would not poison the child because of the protective effect of just the right amount of antitoxin. If this unstable balance was thrown off, however, the child would be exposed to the deadly diphtheria toxin. This approach was abandoned in the 1920s, but not before there were many deaths.

Between October 23 and November 13, 1919, the city of Dallas Health Department injected over 300 children with TAM. Of these, 120 children became ill. There was burning at the injection site initially, then later agonizing pain and swelling of the injected arm. This progressed to massive edema until the skin literally burst open. There was high fever, vomiting, and then signs of heart failure and paralysis. At the site of the injection there was "a ragged, ill-smelling, gangrenous mass of tissue..." Ten children died; the survivors had a long convalescence.

BUNDABERG DISASTER, 1928

Bundaberg in Queensland, Australia, is a seaside city of about 43,000 residents. It is best known for its natural beauty, especially the coral reefs. Only a few elders remember the disaster of 1928. Diphtheria was rampant in those days, and many, even most, families lost at least one child to the deadly infection, so the advent of a vaccine was welcome. On January 12, 1928, some twenty-one children received the vaccine. Within five to twenty hours they became violently ill with fever, rash, vomiting, diarrhea, and loss of consciousness. Twelve died. The vaccine itself was not to blame, but it had become contaminated with staph bacteria, which was the probable cause of the deaths. In retrospect the clinical picture closely resembles TSS (toxic shock syndrome), which we today equate in the public mind with tampon use.

ST. LOUIS, MISSOURI, 1901

In 1901, diphtheria antiserum was derived from the serum of horses that had been immunized with diphtheria toxin. The particular horse in this episode was named Jim, who had some fame because of his high output of antibodies. Unfortunately he became infected with tetanus. Before he developed symptoms of tetanus, his blood was drawn to prepare the usual diphtheria antiserum. There was no way of knowing that Jim's blood already contained tetanus toxin, and for some reason the usual animal toxicity tests were not done on the incriminated batch of serum. In October of that year, twenty unfortunate children who received the diphtheria antiserum contaminated with tetanus toxin became ill.... Fourteen died the particularly horrible death of tetanus—lockjaw.

A special commission was established to investigate the disaster. They found that the "Conditions in the city laboratory were very irregular." Thus a treatment to prevent one disease—diphtheria—caused an even worse one, tetanus.

KYOTO, JAPAN, 1948

In October 1948, more than 15,000 babies and children in Kyoto were injected with a diphtheria toxoid vaccine. Of these, 606 became ill. No fewer than sixty-eight died. Again, the deaths were due to diphtheria toxin not fully neutralized. The symptoms were much like those in the Dallas disaster.

YELLOW FEVER I: AVIAN LEUKOSIS, 1960

Yellow fever is a tropical disease caused by a virus that infects many jungle mammals and is transmitted to man by mosquito. In urban areas it is also transmitted by mosquitoes from man to man. The illness begins about a week after the bite and at first resembles a severe case of the flu. Experienced clinicians in the field have learned to suspect the diagnosis when the sick patient has a small pointed tongue bright red on the tip and sides with a white coat in the center. An unusually slow pulse in the presence of high fever is said to be another sign. After a few days the patient begins to feel better; most fully recover. About 15 percent, however, become sick again. This time the disease attacks every internal organ, including blood and bone marrow. Fever and shock and internal bleeding follow. The patient vomits partially digested blood, giving rise to the Black Vomit moniker.

Ultimately the liver is destroyed and the patient turns yellow, from which the name yellow fever derives. Death at that point is inevitable.

Yellow fever appeared in South America at the time of the Spanish conquests in the seventeenth century. It raged unchecked for three hundred years, until the discovery that it is transmitted by mosquitoes. An epidemic occurred in New Orleans in 1878, killing thirteen thousand people in the worst medical disaster of its time. The U.S. government supported yellow fever research in part because during the Spanish-American War of 1898, far more soldiers died of the disease than from combat wounds. It was during the U.S. occupation of Cuba (1898–1902) that members of Walter Reed's group—the Yellow Fever Commission—proved the mosquito theory by letting themselves be bitten by infected mosquitoes. In time Walter Reed became an icon for the self-sacrificing hero, although in fact, on the day of the crucial experiments, he just happened to have an appointment in Washington. Another commission member, physician William Jesse Lazear, died of yellow fever from the sought-after mosquito bite. The experiments convinced skeptics not only of the transmission mode, but also of the need to control mosquitoes.

At the same time, work was going forward on the development of a live virus vaccine. Those efforts were successful, and a highly effective and safe vaccine was approved in the 1930s. It was not until 1966, however, that researchers realized that the vaccine had been contaminated by a bird virus, avian leukosis. Avian leukosis virus causes several different cancers in birds, including of the kidney, bone marrow, and spleen. Alarmingly, a closely related virus causes cancer in mammals.

Many millions, including a third of the World War II armed services personnel, received this vaccine without obvious harm. A government-sponsored study in 1972, however, concluded that "it is certainly plausible that these [cancer producing] viruses may turn out to be more than innocent passengers."[1] A Veterans Administration study published the same year showed no increase in cancers twenty years after immunization. Surprisingly, leukemia, the most likely cancer, is not specifically mentioned.

Even assuming that the virus is harmless to man, it is a close call, and interestingly, this episode is neither taught nor discussed in medical schools, research institutions, or standard textbooks.

YELLOW FEVER II: HEPATITIS, 1942

March 1942 saw the beginning of an epidemic of hepatitis in U.S. army personnel. Fever, nausea, vomiting, and ultimately yellow jaundice affected many thousands and led to the hospitalization of 51,000 during the ensuing seven months. One hundred fifty died during the acute illness; at least twenty-four survivors developed liver cancer many years later, and an undetermined number developed cirrhosis.

The hepatitis emerged fourteen or fifteen weeks after the administration of the yellow fever vaccine. At that time the vaccine contained human blood serum, which carried the hepatitis virus. The human serum in the original vaccine came from medical student volunteers, one of whom was jaundiced at the time of donation. Several others had a history of hepatitis.

Hepatitis B and C were then unknown and, regrettably, there are no blood samples preserved. In 1993, tests done on some of the survivors, however, showed that virtually all had evidence of hepatitis B infection. This disaster is the largest hepatitis epidemic ever recorded. Vaccination of military personnel continues to be an issue today.

LÜBECK DISASTER, 1919

Lübeck is a seaport in the state Schleswig-Holstein in northern Germany. Count Adolf Holstein founded the city in 1143. Twice destroyed by fire (in the twelfth century and again in World War II) and twice rebuilt, it had great renown as a commercial and political center in the Middle Ages. But in the early twentieth century, unfortunately, it was noted most for the "Lübeck disaster."

Tuberculosis was rampant in postindustrial Europe; it was a leading cause of death. In 1919, Albert Calmette, a pupil of Pasteur's, returned to Paris from a five-year sojourn in Saigon. He and a colleague, Camille Guerin, spent the next thirteen years developing a tuberculosis vaccine. They found that the cow tuberculosis bacterium lost its virulence when grown through many generations in a medium containing bile, but could still evoke antibody responses in humans. The earliest vaccines were taken by mouth, but later preparations were given by injection. The vaccine was widely accepted in continental Europe, but the British and the U.S. did not approve its use. As so often has occurred in the history of medicine, new vaccines (indeed new anything) were subject to great controversy.

In the case of the BCG (Bacille Calmette-Guerin), the usual controversy became virtually a war after the Lübeck disaster. In 1929, Calmette received a request for a BCG culture from the director of public health in Lübeck. The culture was sent and the Lübeck labs prepared the vaccine, which was administered to 242 children. Within a few weeks, seventy-two of the children were dead of overwhelming tuberculosis. Many of the surviving children had late complications, including cirrhosis of the liver. The symptoms were gruesome. Since this was an oral vaccine, most of the symptoms began with diarrhea, fever, nausea, and projectile vomiting due to bowel obstruction. Glands in the neck grew to hen's size, choking off the airway. The children became wasted, and many had brain damage due to tubercles meningitis.

Calmette was vilified and ridiculed until an extensive investigation found that the Lübeck lab directors had accidentally contaminated the cultures with virulent human tuberculosis bacteria. Both directors, Dr. Georg Deycke and Dr. Ernst Alstaedt, were accused of manslaughter by negligence. "The long-drawn-out spectacle of the trial resembled an ancient Greek tragedy, played between the doctors and the fates, pursuing its way relentlessly to its climax of horror and death, and watched by a crowd of parents who served as the chorus, uttering their dismay...." The story was heard all over Europe.

The two were convicted of criminal behavior and sentenced to prison for twenty-four and fifteen months respectively. A subsequent trial exonerated the BCG vaccine, which was later used extensively worldwide.

SV40, 1950

The weekend train rides in the country to visit my brother in the polio hospital were a treat for me. There were picnic tables on the grounds, and my father always brought along a big thermos bottle of hot chocolate. My brother had become ill in the July heat of 1945, an era of summertime panic, when annual epidemics of paralytic polio disrupted life and society. Polio was the AIDS of the first half of the twentieth century, worse even because it spared no class or group. Many recovered, as did my brother, but other survivors were left crippled or dependent on life support. It was the time of the iron lung, infantile paralysis, Sister Kenney, and the March of Dimes.

So when the Salk vaccine was licensed ten years later, it was enthusiastically embraced. Between 1955 and 1963, as many as 10 million people, mostly children, were immunized. What no one knew at the time was that in addition to the lifesaving vaccine, the recipients were also receiving a dose of a live monkey virus, now known as SV40, the fortieth known monkey (simian) virus.

The polio vaccine was prepared from cultures of rhesus monkey kidneys. These monkeys, genetically close to humans, are often infected with the SV40 virus, which does not harm the monkeys. The virus, undetected in the manufacturing process, contaminated many batches of vaccine, both oral and injectable.

The story of the discovery of this contamination is, unfortunately, an oft-repeated tale of bureaucratic rigidity and control. In 1960, Bernice Eddy,[2] on her own initiative, tested monkey kidney cell extracts for cancer-causing agents. She injected the extract into newborn hamsters, many of which developed tumors. These results, which were never allowed to be published, were met with scorn or indifference. Unintimidated, Dr. Eddy disclosed her findings in an unscheduled presentation at a scientific meeting. She was promptly taken off polio vaccine safety testing and prohibited from submitting her work for publication. But the issue was taken up by Merck researchers, who ultimately isolated and identified the SV40 virus.

The SV40 virus is a type of virus that causes cancer, as it did in Dr. Eddy's hamsters. The virus "immortalizes" human cells in culture, indicating a malignant potential. The virus has been found in several kinds of human cancers, including brain, mesothelioma lung cancers, and a highly malignant form of bone cancer. SV40 is a close relative of the JC virus, which attacks the brains of immunosuppressed hosts. It is also a close relative of the SIV-monkey AIDS virus.

SV40 appears to have a strong foothold in the population. One study found evidence of SV40 infection in as many as 23 percent of individuals. Mysteriously, this includes persons too young to have received the contaminated vaccine. SV40 is present in children today. The CDC interprets this to mean that SV40 is a naturally acquired infection not caused by the vaccine. A more likely explanation is that the persons infected by the vaccine have transmitted the virus from person to person or on to the next generation vertically from parent to child. SV40 has been found in semen, providing one established mechanism. The implications of this are, obviously, that any SV40 problems may not, as has been hoped, fade away with time. There is even now, ironically, work being done to provide a vaccine against SV40.

How dangerous is SV40? A government-sponsored study concluded that, "It is premature to discuss or speculate on the potential role of SV40 in the development of human cancer."[3] That was 1976; since then there have been plenty of data to "discuss or speculate on." Before looking at some of that data, remember, association does not prove causation. Red automobiles have more accidents, but not because they are red.

In children whose mothers received the possibly contaminated polio vaccine during pregnancy, there was a twofold increase in neurological cancers.[4]

The most alarming data, however, pertain to SV40 and mesothelioma, a cancer arising from the lining of the chest, abdominal, and pericardial cavities. Injection of SV40 material induces mesothelioma in animals. In humans this tumor is an aggressive, lethal cancer; survival for more than a year is rare. The tumor was almost unknown before the second half of the twentieth century, but now causes more than two thousand deaths per year in the United States. Finland conducted a vaccination program much like ours, but their vaccine was free of SV40, and there was no rise in mesothelioma cases during the same time period.

The presence of SV40 has been found in 60 percent of mesotheliomas.[5] Asbestosis is also often associated with mesothelioma, and it appears that either agent or both together may cause this cancer. SV40 is also associated with a variety of brain and other cancers. Researchers in the United States, Germany, Italy, France, and Japan have independently found SV40 in brain tumors. Japanese workers have identified SV40 in bone cancers.

More recently, the prestigious journal *The Lancet* published in a report that researchers have found SV40 in non–Hodgkin's lymphoma variety of cancer. In a commentary on the article,[6] Dr. Malkin states that present studies are sufficient to meet Koch's postulates, which have been used as proof of causality for over a hundred years. The postulates are:

1. A specific microorganism is always associated with a given disease.
2. The microorganism can be isolated from the diseased animal and grown in pure culture in the laboratory.
3. The cultured microbe will cause disease when transferred to a healthy animal.
4. The same type of microorganism can be isolated from the newly infected animal.

In Dr. Malkin's opinion, SV40 has passed the test: It causes cancer in humans.

These arguments have been challenged. The number of cases in most of the reports is small; the tests used to identify the presence of SV40 are prone to inaccuracy; the epidemiological, population-based studies are subject to biases; association does not prove causation. Furthermore, it is unusual for one virus to cause multiple types of tumors, as does SV40. There is some evidence that SV40 has been present in humans since before the polio vaccine era, raising the possibility that human infection with SV40 is a phenomenon of nature unrelated to the vaccine.

Vaccine advocates, including the CDC, FDA, and pediatric societies, minimize the dangers and emphasize the benefits of the polio vaccine. Vaccine opponents do the opposite.

Here is my opinion. SV40 infection was introduced into the human population through the early polio vaccines. The infection has become firmly established by person-to-person contact or mother-to-fetus transmission. This means that the problem will not go away. SV40 is at the very least a cofactor in the genesis of mesothelioma. Its role in other cancers needs further investigation, not a cover-up. The government went ahead with the mandatory polio vaccination program even after discovery of the SV40 contamination. The logic of the decision was that more would die from polio infection than from the then apparently harmless SV infection. So the SV40 news was suppressed. And it is still being suppressed, or at least neglected. Even now there is no commercially available test for SV40. An informal survey of my students and residents found that only 10 percent of them had even heard of SV40. It is high time to aggressively search out the implications of SV40 infection.

THE CUTTER INCIDENT, 1955

It was the spring of 1955. The Salk polio vaccine, an inactivated (killed) whole virus preparation, had been tested on hundreds of thousands of volunteers and was declared safe and effective. Its licensure was welcomed with jubilation and effusive rhetoric. It was called the greatest achievement of medical science; it was the beginning of the end of the terrible summer epidemics. Only a few idiosyncratic critics expressed concern about safety. Hardly anyone referred to the disastrous failure of the 1930s Kolmer and Brodie vaccines, which were far too virulent for clinical use. Salk was lionized, and a world of clinics and vaccination programs were mobilized, with many photo-ops for local officials. This machinery was so effective that in a ten-day period in mid-April, four hundred thousand grade school children were inoculated.

On April 25, less than two weeks after the release of the vaccine, an infant with paralytic poliomyelitis was admitted to the Michael Reese Hospital in Chicago. This case was like the distant rumble of approaching thunder, for the infant had been inoculated in the buttock nine days before. Both legs were paralyzed. Before the awful implications were fully grasped, five similar cases were reported to the California Health Department. All the patients became ill four to ten days after inoculation, and all had paralysis of the inoculated arm.

An investigation by frantic Public Health Service epidemiologists quickly uncovered a connection between these cases and vaccines prepared by Cutter Laboratories. Two days after the first case, Cutter was requested to recall all of its vaccine.

Meanwhile, an ominous event was unfolding. About two weeks after the first wave of cases, a second, larger wave was occurring, this time among household contacts of the original cases. There could be but only one explanation: The Cutter vaccine contained live, virulent polio virus, which infected the original recipients, who were now infecting their family members as well as some in the community.

All immunization was discontinued while the investigation proceeded. The suspicion that at least some of the Cutter batches contained live virus was quickly confirmed. The formaldehyde treatment step, which was supposed to inactivate the virus, had failed to do so. This may have been due to unforeseen changes between laboratory and mass-produced vaccines. In any case, the Cutter vaccine contained clumps of virus that were not fully penetrated by the formaldehyde. The fix seemed easy: a few more tests, the incorporation of superfine filtration, and the problem were solved. Not appreciated at the time, these corrective measures, while increasing the safety of the vaccine, decreased its potency, making it a less effective vaccine.

The Cutter epidemic was soon contained, and by the end of June there were no more cases. Except among the 460 infected children and their families, the "Cutter incident" was soon forgotten.

"ATYPICAL" MEASLES, 1960s

This is about a vaccine that not only didn't work, but made an illness worse. At the time that the live measles vaccine was licensed in 1963, a killed measles vaccine was also released. This had the advantage of being free from the ever present dangers associated with live vaccines. Tested on children, the killed vaccine showed that there was a brisk antibody response with minimal side effects. It was therefore widely used, especially in Canada. At first all seemed well. But within a year or two, measles cases began to crop up in immunized children, and there were reports of isolated epidemics. The vaccine was not preventing measles. Studies done in 1965 explained what was happening. The antibodies rapidly disappeared so that by one year later most children were no longer protected, even after booster doses. But there was much worse news to come. In 1967, Vincent A. Fulginiti, a much-published pediatrician at the University of Colorado in Denver, reported on a series of children who contracted measles five years after vaccination.[7] Ten of these children had a "new disease termed atypical measles." The children had a high fever lasting four to seven days, during which time they had headache, muscle pain, and severe pneumonia, pleurisy, and a "peculiar rash that began on the...ankles and feet and extends towards the trunk." They were ill enough to require hospitalization, but recovered. Numerous similar cases have been published. Another feature of this new disease is that children who received live measles vaccine after being immunized with killed vaccine developed violent reactions to the live vaccine.

It is theorized that the killed vaccine somehow sensitized the children to the measles virus so that they then developed atypical measles when exposed to measles virus vaccine. In a great understatement, Fulginiti wrote, "It is our conclusion that no healthy child should electively receive killed-measles-vaccine." By then an estimated 1.8 million doses had been administered. The vaccine was withdrawn, and the new disease disappeared.

JORDAN, 1998

On September 28, 1998, the annual Jordanian process of immunizing children began, coincident with the start of the school year. The epidemic started the next day when two boys came to school, complained of being dizzy and headachy, and then fainted. The staff became alarmed and called for help. With the arrival of health officers and ambulances, twenty more fainted and were sent to the hospital by ambulance. Soon thereafter TV cameras, newspaper reporters, and police arrived. News of the "bad vaccine" spread like wildfire, and the students fell like bowling pins. By the end of the day, eighty students were hospitalized and by the end of the next day a total of 122. All had been vaccinated with a well-established Td vaccine. All were back home within twenty-four hours, and none died or had any complications.

Although the title of the WHO report[8] implicates mass hysteria or other undefined "psychogenic illness," the data provided suggests otherwise. All the children affected had received the vaccine the day before; no child who did not get vaccine was affected. One batch of vaccine was associated with more cases than other batches. Of the first fifty-five children, 58 percent had fever, 15 percent had chest tightness and "needed oxygen," and 13 percent had transient EKG abnormalities. Most of the symptoms were quite mild and of the type often associated with this type of immunization. One or two children with these symptoms would not have aroused much concern.

On the other hand, it appears that an initial panic by the staff led to a series of administrative decisions and inaccurate news accounts that did contribute a psychogenic component to the incident. This is further supported by the observation that in several instances numerous children became ill almost at the very same moment; this is biologically implausible. One can only conclude that a physiologic adverse vaccine reaction was intensified by psychosocial factors.

CHINA, 2002

Japanese encephalitis is a mosquito-borne viral illness very common in Asia. Although the majority of infections cause no symptoms or a flulike illness, a small percentage of infected individuals (mostly children) develop encephalitis, which causes fever, vomiting, seizures, and paralysis. Many die; survivors are often left with brain damage.

China has an active immunization program, which apparently recently went awry. In the city of Mishan, in a province noted for its agriculture, 8,300 children ages seven through sixteen received the killed-virus Japanese encephalitis vaccine. A WHO spokesperson said that the outbreak was psychogenic in origin. "Around 70 children were hospitalized," but none had abnormal clinical findings.

However, according to a Reuters report, 900 children were hospitalized, and some of the students were seriously ill. Both reports indicate that some heart "irregularities" or "infection" had occurred. Furthermore, the director of the Mishan Epidemic Prevention Center and a deputy chief of the City Education Bureau were arrested and charged with negligence. This does not sound like "mass hysteria."

Enraged parents massed in front of city hall to protest, parents who were particularly incensed about this incident because they have been long subjected to a one-child policy. Any threat to their children elicits a very strong response.

This may turn out to be one of the worst vaccine disasters, but it will be a long time, if ever, before the world knows what happened.

SWINE FLU FIASCO, 1976

During the cold winter of 1976, an epidemic of respiratory infections affected some five hundred soldiers at Fort Dix, New Jersey. Among them was nineteen-year-old Pvt. David Lewis of Ashley Falls, Massachusetts, who elected to leave his sickbed to go on a forced march on February 4. The next day he was critically ill, and he died within twenty-four hours. Four days later the cause of death was determined to be a flu virus variant that closely resembled the devastating strain that caused the 1918 pandemic in which 20 million worldwide and 500,000 in the U.S. died. Twelve other cases were found at Fort Dix; four were hospitalized, but David Lewis was the only fatality. Most of the other soldiers who had come to sick call had a "garden variety" flu infection.

The possibility of another "1918" alarmed health officials, but there were no cases except for the ones at Fort Dix. Some experts took the position that even though there was as yet no epidemic, there was sufficient risk to justify an immunization campaign. Others argued that an epidemic was unlikely because it was late in the flu season; there had been no spread outside of Fort Dix; most of the Fort Dix cases were mild illnesses. They recommended a wait-and-see policy. A middle-of-the-road suggestion was that vaccine be prepared and stockpiled, but not administered, in the absence of an epidemic.

The CDC ultimately took a "better safe than sorry" approach and recommended a national swine flu immunization policy. The decision, although wrong, was rational and reasonable. What followed was not.

The CDC presented President Ford with a $136 million plan to immunize every man, woman, and child. The media jumped on the issue and big headlines and scare stories were the meat of the day. On March 24, during primetime the day after a surprise loss to Reagan in the North Carolina Republican presidential primary, the president announced the plan. He was flanked on either side by Salk and Sabin of polio vaccine[9] fame. A memo from the secretary of the Department of Health, Education and Welfare to the Office of Management and Budget indicated "that the projections are that this virus will kill one million Americans in 1976."

The vaccine pharmaceutical manufacturers were under tremendous pressure to create a vaccine "yesterday." The CDC's reputation was on the line; Ronald Reagan was challenging Ford in the upcoming primaries; the public was in an uproar. The tension was not much relieved when the insurance companies refused to provide liability coverage for vaccine manufacturers. The pharmaceutical houses in turn refused to distribute the vaccine without liability protection. The ball passed to Congress, which was reluctant to accept such an open-ended commitment, especially since there was no swine flu in evidence. The political pressure was too strong to resist, however, and Congress ultimately passed the Swine Flu Act of 1976, which provided for the federal government to assume the liability for any vaccine mishaps. Laughably, the bill's passage was, assisted by the propitious occurrence of the Philadelphia Legionnaire epidemic, which was initially attributed to swine flu.

The frantically prepared first batch of swine flu vaccine produced by one pharmaceutical house produced no antibodies to swine flu. The CDC had given the manufacturer the wrong strain of flu virus. Two million worthless doses were discarded. The virus grew slowly, so that production goals had to be halved. Subsequent batches produced adequate antibody levels only when large doses that produced frequent side effects were used.

Finally, on October 1 the program was gotten underway. On October 12, three elderly persons in Pittsburgh, Pennsylvania, died on the same day within hours after receiving swine flu shots. Pennsylvania and several other states suspended the program. The CDC came to its defense, and President Ford and his family got their "shots" on television. The program was resumed, but by this time the swine flu nonepidemic had become a joke, and Ford's commitment to the program was known as "Flugate" in contrast to the Watergate of his predecessor.

By the end of November, however, the laughter disappeared as reports started coming in of people suffering serious neurological damage after receiving the flu vaccine. Patients were coming down with GBS (Guillain-Barre syndrome),[10] also known as acute inflammatory demyelinating polyneuropathy, or Landry's ascending paralysis. Jean Baptiste Octave Landry de Thezillat's description written in 1859 cannot be bettered:

> The sensory and motor systems may be equally affected. However, the main problem is usually a motor disorder characterized by a gradual diminution of muscular strength with flaccid limbs and without contractures, convulsions or reflex movements of any kind. In almost all cases, micturation and defecation remain normal. One does not observe any symptoms referable to the central nervous system, spinal pain or tenderness, headache or delirium. The intellectual faculties are preserved until the end. The onset of the paralysis can be preceded by a general feeling of weakness, pins and needles and even slight cramps. Alternatively the illness may begin suddenly and end unexpectedly. In both cases the weakness spreads rapidly from the lower to the upper parts of the body with a universal tendency to become generalized.
>
> The first symptoms always affect the extremities of the limbs and the lower limbs particularly. When the whole body becomes affected the order of progression is more or less constant: (1) toe and foot muscles, then the hamstrings and glutei, and finally the anterior and adductor muscles of the thigh; (2) finger and hand, arm and then shoulder muscles; (3) trunk muscles; (4) respiratory muscles, tongue, pharynx, oesophagus, etc. The paralysis then becomes generalized but more severe in the distal parts of the extremities. The progression can be more or less rapid. It was eight days in one and fifteen

days in another case which I believe can be classified as acute. More often it is scarcely two or three days and sometimes only a few hours. When the paralysis reaches its maximum intensity the danger of asphyxia is always imminent. However, in eight out of ten cases death was avoided either by skillful professional intervention or a spontaneous remission of this phase of the illness. In two cases death occurred at this stage.... When the paralysis recedes it demonstrates the reverse of the phenomenon which signaled its development. The upper parts of the body, the last to be affected, are the first to recover their mobility which then returns from above downwards.

Death occurs when the muscles of breathing, the diaphragm's and rib cage muscles, become paralyzed. Modern respirators and intensive care can usually keep the patient alive until recovery, which may take months.

GBS is one of the autoimmune diseases; the body's immune system attacks its own tissue. An infection with a virus or, in the case of GBS, administration of a vaccine somehow disorders the immune system so that it no longer recognizes "self" and attacks the victim's own tissues. In the cases of GBS, the nerves are affected.

The GBS epidemic, of course, put an inglorious end to the swine flu immunization program. It was officially halted on December 16, 1976.

The whole affair started with a reasonable concern that a flu pandemic might be in the offing, but the issue was soon overtaken by a deadly mix of uncertain science, politics, pride, hidden agendas, and lots of money.

In the end there were only fifty-three deaths among the 45 million vaccinated. Most of the GBS patients recovered. It could have been much worse.

CHAPTER 4

The Current Controversy: In Perspective

Vaccination is more than one hundred years old and has been controversial from the start. Of all the benefits of medical science, vaccination is at or near the summit. It is also the most controversial of routine medical procedures. There is an antivaccination movement that seeks to stop vaccination, and its arguments cover the spectrum from reasonable discourse to hysterical paranoia. Let us try to understand the opposition.

To begin with, vaccination is counterintuitive. What sense does it make to inject a well baby with a potent, biologically active vaccine that contains elements of the very disease it is supposed to prevent? Vaccination meddles with a core biological function essential to life. I say "meddles with" because the immune system affects every organ and cell and is vastly complicated, but we know very little about it. In many cases, questions about the effect of vaccines are unanswered—and probably through ignorance, unasked.

Some vaccines contain living microbes; the vaccination is literally an infection with a variant of the disease-causing agent. Vaccines contain poisons and chemicals, including mercury, formaldehyde, antibiotics, and aluminum salts. Vaccines also contain material derived from animals, including beef, horse, chick, monkey, and duck.

Many vaccines have been recalled or discontinued because they were toxic or ineffective. The rotavirus and lyme disease vaccines are two recent examples. Some vaccines have serious side effects; children have died. Convulsions, fever, rashes, nerve, and brain damage are some of these "side effects" caused by vaccines.

The antivaccinationists also note, correctly, that the number of cases of common childhood diseases had dropped dramatically in the prevaccine era, and on the other hand, even some vaccinated children get infected. This is taken as evidence that vaccines don't work.

More sophisticated critics are concerned about the age shift caused by vaccines. Natural infection tends to induce lifelong immunity, whereas vaccine-induced immunity tends to wear off. This results in a population of nonimmune adults and, as is well known, many mild childhood diseases are severe in adults.

Under some conditions a good vaccine can make things worse. The rubella syndrome[1] has almost disappeared in the USA because of near universal immunity, thanks to adult booster shots. But where vaccination is spotty, the vaccine may decrease the natural infection rate and so increase the number of susceptibles. The chicken pox vaccine is unnecessary and may cause an epidemic of shingles in years to come.

Medical policymaking is always entwined with politics and financial profits. The medical establishment, the pharmaceutical industry, and political interest groups influence vaccine policies to favor their interests. This whiff of corruption further energizes the antivaccination group. Reinforcing all that resentment is the policy of mandatory vaccination.

So why vaccinate? Vaccination saves millions of lives and prevents a world of suffering. We know that vaccines do work. Epidemiological studies, clinical trials, antibody titers, and recurrence of disease when vaccination is discontinued all prove that vaccines work. None of them work 100 percent of the time; none of them are 100 percent safe. Each vaccine has unique problems and benefits. The reduction in the number of cases before the vaccine era was probably due to better hygiene, antibiotics, and better nutrition. But in all cases the common infections persisted at a lower but still significant level until a vaccine became available. No disease has been known to disappear spontaneously. Now smallpox is gone; polio is not far behind.

The problem of age shift can be addressed by developing longer-lasting vaccines or developing boosters for adults. The concern about autism and the many other unproven toxicities is usually due to confusion about causality and coincidence. Autism typically starts at the age when immunizations are routinely administered, so of course the two appear to be related, but are not. As for late toxicity appearing years after vaccination, this remains to be seen.

The mercury story is complicated but moot in the USA because there is no longer mercury in the routine vaccines. The other chemicals, and animal products, are in trace amounts and harmless.

Sometimes a vaccine is a victim of its own success. As the disease disappears, the side effects alone remain. Today's parents have never seen the horror of whooping cough or the grisly death of tetanus, so their tolerance of vaccine side effects approaches zero.

The controversy gets really hot when the issue is vaccine injury. How many infections or deaths prevented justify a death from a vaccine? Some would say it is never justified; better a thousand cases of measles than the life of one healthy child. Peggy Omar[2] even goes so far as to write, "It is immoral to risk the health of even one child in order to save the lives of many." To the medical scientist such a position is illogical, inhibits further medical advances, and denies children the freedom to grow up healthy.

The pro and anti sides of the debate, having staked opposing positions based on mutually exclusive premises, will likely stand across another hundred years of controversy.

PART 2

The Common Vaccines

CHAPTER 5

Smallpox Vaccine

A study of smallpox is virtually a study of modern man and his civilization, for smallpox has been with us for thousands of years and is with us still, and so are our attempts to control it. Science and superstition, charity and cruelty, politics, wars, human suffering, and the fate of peoples are intertwined in this history. The smallpox vaccine story is especially interesting because it pits modern medicine against folk remedies, practitioners against professors, charlatans against scientists.

Most histories of smallpox (and there have been many) begin with the Jenner myth. According to this myth, Edward Jenner, a selfless country doctor, noticed that most faces, especially in the city, bore the scars of smallpox, but the cheeks of the fair milkmaids were unblemished. He postulated that the frequent occurrence of cowpox on the hands of these women protected them somehow from smallpox. To prove his theory, Jenner performed an experiment. On May 14, 1796, he took a sample of pus from a festering cowpox ulcer on the hand of Blossom's milkmaid, Sarah Nelmes, and administered it to young Master James Phipps. Then, on July 1, Jenner attempted to inoculate James with fully virulent smallpox. The inoculations failed to take, indicating that James was immune to smallpox. Jenner termed this procedure "vaccination" after the Latin word for cow. The vaccination had succeeded. Jenner made no secret of this initial success, and, although there were many skeptics, other practitioners joined the ranks of vaccinationists.

The myth is neat. The truth is messy. As we noted in an earlier chapter, variolation had been practiced for hundreds of years before Jenner's time. Jenner knew that although dangerous, a person could be protected from severe smallpox by deliberately inducing a mild case. It was also no secret that farmer Benjamin Jetsy, using a stocking needle, had inoculated his wife and two sons with cowpox twenty years earlier, with good results. Mrs. Jetsy lived to be eighty-four.

Far from being selfless, Jenner was always a strong advocate of himself, using personal connections and financial backing of wealthy friends to secure priority for his discovery and publications. He was also more thorough in reporting his successes than in noting failures and complications, of which there were many, including the transmission of syphilis.

These are old issues that dull the luster but do not destroy the myth. Some recent scholarship, however, raises issues that are more serious.[1] Razzel's thesis is that most of Jenner's vaccine was a modified smallpox virus, not cowpox. We have already seen how easy it is for a vaccine to become contaminated. In Jenner's day it was easier still. The study of infectious disease was just beginning. The only way Jenner could tell if a vaccine contained cowpox or smallpox was by the symptoms. Cowpox inoculations caused a painful ulcer; smallpox caused blisters sometimes at a distance from the inoculations. However, sometimes the cowpox inoculations did not "take," and sometimes a weak smallpox reaction looked like a cowpox reaction. The vaccine was prepared by soaking a thread in the cowpox "matter" and letting it dry. Others, including Woodville, Pearson, and Waterhouse, also prepared vaccines. In times of plenty, they freely shared their threads with comrades and colleagues. At times, however, a good case of cowpox was hard to come by, and the only way to propagate the vaccine was "from arm-to-arm." Such serial passage is a good way to weaken a virus, and it was probably such an attenuated smallpox virus that Jenner sent to Waterhouse in Marblehead, Massachusetts, in July 1800. At the time there was no smallpox in the community. At first the inoculations went well, although the formation of blisters in some cases was of some concern. Later, in October, several individuals had severe reactions, and by the end of the month the unfortunate town was the site of a smallpox epidemic, which killed sixty-eight people. An attenuated virus sometimes reverts to virulence, as probably happened at Marblehead.

Where does this leave Jenner? Myths can never be proven wrong, and perhaps in this case it is just as well. Except for the Marblehead piece, the myth makes a good story, and Jenner did, after all, do more than any man of his time to advance the practice of immunization.

Smallpox vaccines today contain vaccinia, a virus cousin of smallpox and cowpox, but distinct from both. Its origin is lost in the haze of history. Many different stains of vaccinia have been cultured. Some of the vaccinia strains have been grown in rabbits, chickens, water buffalo, and other animals. The most commonly used strains today are the New York City

Board of Health strain (New York) and the Temple of Heaven strain (China), both grown in calfskin.

As we will see in a later chapter, there have always been groups strongly opposed to vaccination in general and smallpox immunization in particular because it involves deliberately infecting a human with an animal virus.

In spite of the objections, it is clear that vaccination is highly successful in preventing smallpox. So successful, in fact, that in 1980, WHO pronounced the world free of smallpox. This singular accomplishment, the actual eradication of a dread disease that had plagued humankind for thousands of years, was hailed as the greatest achievement of medical science. As late as 1999, the definitive text on vaccination[2] opens the smallpox chapter with the statement that "Smallpox is now a disease of historical interest only...."

In a world free of smallpox there is no need for a vaccine, especially one that sometimes has serious side effects, so vaccination was discontinued worldwide by 1985. The result is that almost everyone on earth today is susceptible to smallpox.[3] In the preeradication days, there was always a population of smallpox survivors who were immune to further infection. These individuals served as a kind of firewall to limit spread of the infection. They no longer exist. Reintroduction of wild smallpox virus could cause perhaps the worst epidemic in history.

The hot smallpox topic in the 1970s was whether to destroy the existing smallpox cultures. Officially, only the CDC in Atlanta and the Research Institute for Viral Preparations (known as Vector) in Novosibirsk, Siberia, were allowed to keep smallpox cultures. Arguments favoring destruction of the world's remaining smallpox virus include the prevention of accidental release of the virus into the environment, prevention of the use of smallpox as a terrorist weapon, and the final elimination of smallpox. Counterarguments are that CIA reports indicate that multiple stocks of live virus already exist in unauthorized locations including North Korea, China, Pakistan, Israel, Iraq, Iran, and Cuba.[4] Moreover, even if all the laboratory cultures were destroyed, smallpox could reappear by natural mechanisms such as the preservation of the virus in individuals who died in the permafrost or through a virulent mutation of another pox virus. More compelling is the argument that there is so much to learn about viruses and their interaction with humans that preservation of live virus is crucial for research purposes. Some even argue that deliberately destroying a natural life form—smallpox virus—is unethical.

These discussions were swept off the table by the rising concern about smallpox as a biological weapon if we were to invade Iraq. In December

2002, Bush personally announced his plan for mass vaccination against smallpox. CNN quoted him as saying, "As commander in chief, I do not believe I can ask others to accept this risk unless I am willing to do the same. Therefore I will receive the vaccine along with our military."[5] The plan called for immediate mandatory vaccination of 500,000 military personnel. This was to be followed by vaccination of 440,000 health care workers. The next phase was to immunize 10 million "first responders," mainly staffs of medical facilities, rescue workers, and police. Licensed vaccine was to be available to the public in 2004.

By April 2003, about four months after the announcement of this grandiose plan, it was a failure and no one wanted to even mention it.

The plan was flawed in its essence, which was the assumption that universal immunization would do more good than harm. Critics of the program pointed to the historical data: two deaths per million doses, up to fifty-two serious, life-threatening complications per million doses; and 900 less severe reactions such as fever, rash, and scarring. Among these are generalized vaccinia, in which the patient is overwhelmed by the live vaccine. This occurs most often to individuals who have impaired immunity. The number of such individuals has increased since smallpox vaccination was discontinued, thanks to HIV, chemotherapy, and cancer.

Additional considerations included the fact that there was not enough vaccine available (although there was some evidence that the vaccine could be diluted up to five times and still be effective). The vaccine that was available was over twenty years old and had been supposedly cautiously frozen. The pharmaceutical industry was charged with the development of a safer, cheaper vaccine that could rapidly be manufactured in large quantities. The industry's enthusiasm was limited by liability concerns if (as seemed likely) an individual suffered harm from the old or yet-to-be-licensed new vaccines. Accordingly, the Homeland Security Act of 2002, Section 304, was amended to protect medical and pharmaceutical entities from lawsuits.

The risk of nationwide vaccination outweighed the risk of nonexistent smallpox infection. Epidemiologists, clinicians, administrators, and knowledgeable legislators opposed the plan, but President Bush pushed on. Physicians, hospitals, and state governments[6] refused to participate.

The result was that the vaccination rate was far below the original estimate. The program limped along, however, until reports of heart disease began to come in from the field. Smallpox vaccine has been used for a hundred years without any hint of heart disease. But one recent paper (Harness) describes 140 cases of inflammation of the heart muscle and the covering of the heart (myopericarditis), occurring up to thirty days after smallpox vaccination. The early cases were extensively publicized, and an already wary population wanted no part of the smallpox vaccine. The whole program quietly tiptoed into oblivion, leaving puzzled medical scientists trying to understand how a new side effect came into being.

Smallpox was eradicated in 1980, but it is with us still.

CHAPTER 6

Chicken Pox Vaccine

Does the world need a chicken pox vaccine? The manufacturer (Merck) of the vaccine thinks so. The web page http://www.info.com/menu.htm. shows a beautiful mother and adorable child under the caption "I never realized chickenpox could be so serious," also "...infections result in 'flesh-eating' disease." The National Immunization Program's website (http://www.cdc.gov/nip/diseases/varicella/) warns, "It's more serious than you think" in giant yellow letters.

However, another point of view is captured by an anonymous clinician: "Chicken pox is most commonly an annoying illness lasting three to seven days, and happily never seen again."

VZV, Varicella zoster virus, causes chicken pox and shingles. Varicella, the Latin name for chicken pox, is a diminutive form of variola, also known as smallpox. Some believe that "chicken" pox derives from the Old English word *gican*, which means "itch" and is pronounced with a soft g. Most authorities, however, believe that the allusion is to the chickpea, *pois chiche* in French. When sliced in half and laid on a pink-colored disc, the chickpea bears a remarkable resemblance to the characteristic blisters seen in chicken pox.[1]

The point is that smallpox and chicken pox were not distinguished from each other until 1767, when William Heberden's[2] clinical observations made clear the difference. Unlike the sores of chicken pox, smallpox lesions start in the extremities and move to the trunk and head. The lesions are all of the same age, whereas chicken pox lesions occur in several crops.

Before 1995, when the chicken pox vaccine was licensed in the USA, we all had chicken pox whether we knew it or not. Everyone was familiar with the spots that appear out of nowhere or are preceded by a mild fever for two to three days. The spots, as many as five hundred, start on the scalp, spread to face and trunk and then to the limbs. They develop into fragile blisters that break, then scab over and heal. Sometimes there are no spots or rash at all, but blood tests may show that the infection definitely occurred. Over 90 percent of nonimmune household contacts will catch the disease. These secondary cases are usually more severe than the original. Chicken pox in general appears to produce lifelong immunity, but occasionally chicken pox occurs a second time. These recurrences are milder than natural infection.

Serious complications and deaths do occur. In the USA, before the vaccine, there were about a hundred deaths per year. These were due to the chicken pox virus itself or, more often, secondary bacterial infections. Chicken pox is most severe in adults, in children less than one year old, and in persons who have a depressed immune system.

The most common complication is bacterial infection of the open sores. Especially lethal is the streptococcus germ (the "flesh-eating bacteria" of the excitable media). Viral pneumonia due to the chicken pox virus occurs almost exclusively in adults and carries a 50 percent mortality. The characteristic chest x-ray shows a blizzard of shadows affecting all of both lungs. Rare neurologic complications include inflammation of various parts of the brain, causing a spectrum of symptoms including irritability, slurred speech, loss of balance, meningitis, and, rarely, death.

Individuals who have severe immunosuppression may have "progressive varicella." The virus overcomes bodily defenses and fatally attacks the internal organs, including the liver and brain. Concern for this disaster was the driving force for the development of the chicken pox vaccine.

Natural chicken pox infection creates immunological pandemonium. Antibodies, white cells, killer cells, and kinins all join in to attack the invading virus. When the peace treaty is finally signed, the patient is well but the virus is only under house arrest and lying dormant and inactive in the nerves near the spinal cord, to which it has retreated. When the conditions are ripe, the virus may become reactivated, but then the resulting illness is shingles.

SHINGLES

Shingles, also known as Herpes zoster, is caused by the chicken pox virus. *Herpes* is Greek for "to creep." The terms *zoster* and *shingles* derive from the respective Greek and Latin terms *zoster* and *cingulum,* for the "girdle"-like distribution of the rash.

Reactivation of the dormant VZV is most likely if the immune system is weak, as occurs in the elderly and in AIDS, cancer, chemotherapy, and post–organ transplant patients. A drop in antibodies with the passage of time may be another critical factor.

The shingles patient develops a blistery rash that is usually confined to a band across one side of the chest, back, or limbs. Shingles may also affect the head and face. It is restricted to the right or left side of the body, not crossing the midline. The patient, usually over fifty years old, experiences itch and pain that may precede the rash by days. The alert clinician may make the diagnosis before the telltale rash appears. The rash clears up in several days, but unfortunately the pain may last for days or even weeks and months. The pain is unremitting, sometimes intense, and does not much diminish, even with strong painkillers. Insomnia, depression, and weight loss may destroy the fabric of the patient's life. Chronic pain clinics always have a complement of these patients with their "post-herpetic syndrome."

Perhaps even worse is the blindness due to the aggressive inflammation caused by shingles affecting the eye. Invasion of nerves in the face may cause facial paralysis and shingles in the ear. Fortunately, these disasters are uncommon.

We do not know what effect the chicken pox vaccine will have on the frequency and severity of shingles.

THE VACCINE

There are many manufacturers of chicken pox vaccine, each with a unique combination of components, but all contain live viruses derived from the Oka strain of chicken pox virus. This strain was isolated in the 1970s from a chicken pox blister on a three-year-old child in Japan, of family name Oka. The virus was attenuated by growing it in the cold and having it make multiple passes through human fetal tissue and various animal[3] cells. The results of the animal testing were encouraging.

As the number of transplant and chemotherapy patients increased, progressive varicella took an increasing toll from these immunosuppressed children. In the USA, 30 percent of children with leukemia who got chicken pox became severely ill, and 7 percent died. Interest in a vaccine was intense all over the world. Japanese scientists were the first to develop a vaccine, derived from the Oka strain.

Although the rule is to not give a live vaccine to immunosuppressed individuals, researchers found that under tightly controlled conditions, the children could tolerate the vaccine and did develop immunity: The vaccine was effective. Based on these studies, the use of the vaccine was expanded to "at-risk" nonimmune adults, including health care workers, teachers, and nonimmune parents of young children. Multiple clinical studies have shown the vaccine to be safe and effective. Accordingly, in 1995, ACIP[4] and the American Academy of Pediatrics advocated universal immunization for children twelve months to twelve years old; younger and older children are more likely to have side effects.

Efficacy in preventing chicken pox approaches 90 percent, even when put to the most stringent test: protection of nonimmune persons in a household exposed to an active case. Some "breakthrough" cases do occur, but they are always mild.

The chicken pox vaccine is safe. Soreness at the injection site is common, as may be a low-grade transient fever and irritability. About 3 percent of vaccinees will have a mild rash or a few blisters. The vaccine virus can be transmitted within the family, but this happens rarely, and when it does happen it results in a very mild rash.

The vaccine is in powder form and is reconstituted by dissolving it in a special fluid provided by the manufacturer. The vaccine is fragile and must be kept frozen.

THE CONTROVERSY

Universal chicken pox immunization has been controversial from the first. Advocates point out correctly that the vaccine is safe and effective. Without a vaccine, 90 percent of the population becomes infected, so the number of cases per year is the same as the number of births per year, which is about 3.8 million. The vaccine would prevent a world of itching and anxiety; prevent 300,000 cases of chicken pox, 650 cases of encephalitis, and 380 deaths per year. Furthermore, several studies have shown that using the vaccine would save money if one takes into account wages lost by parents kept home from work, the cost of medications prescribed for the sick children, and the cost of their medical care, including office visits.

Based on these considerations, the government recommends universal childhood vaccination. Opponents argue that vaccinations are not necessary. The complications of chicken pox are rare, and some of the "chicken pox" deaths are due to underlying leukemia or immune suppression. Chicken pox encephalitis is very mild and short-lived in 97 percent of cases. The argument for universal vaccination as a way to save money raises some sticky questions about values. Furthermore, the cost/benefit analysis is a mathematical stretch based on untestable assumptions.[5] If, as seems likely, an additional booster is required, or if shingles cases increase, any theoretical cost savings will disappear.

A major issue is the effect the chicken pox vaccine will have on the age of persons acquiring natural chicken pox. Chicken pox is life-threatening in infants under one year old and in adults. Naturally, acquired chicken pox usually does not occur in the first year of life because of the mother's antibodies; it does not usually occur in adults because almost all are immune from having had childhood chicken pox.

If most but not all children are vaccinated, the unvaccinated ones may become adults who are susceptible to chicken pox. In the case of women of childbearing age, susceptibility to chicken pox is triply bad. The mother is at risk of getting adult chicken pox. The fetus is at risk of congenital abnormalities or death. Additionally, the infant is deprived of the mother's anti–chicken pox antibodies, which protect it in that vulnerable first year.

Even if there were 100 percent vaccination, the problem of age shift would remain if, as seems likely, vaccine-induced immunity wears off with time. Everyone knows that chicken pox rarely occurs twice because having it once makes you immune for life. What not everyone knows is that this lifelong immunity may be the result of repeated contact with the chicken pox virus, causing a bump in antibody levels but no symptoms. If the vaccine eliminates these bumps, more adults will be susceptible. In this respect, the less effective the vaccine, the better.[6] Natural infection produces antibody levels much higher than does vaccination. Lower antibodies mean less solid protection. Furthermore, vaccine-induced antibodies probably do not last as long as natural antibodies.[7]

The only way around this problem of age shift caused by vaccination is 100 percent universal chicken pox vaccination so that the virus is no longer in the environment. This will be a long time in coming, if ever. An alternative is to provide booster shots to adolescents and adults. However, there is no licensed vaccine for them because of the high rate of side effects. There are adult vaccines in development, but they will surely have unique problems of their own.

Next comes the shingles problem. As we have seen, shingles occurs when the dormant VZV virus becomes active because of a falloff of immunity due to disease, medication, or old age. What effect will the chicken pox vaccine have on shingles? According to Brisson,[8] "Mass varicella vaccination is expected to cause a major epidemic of herpes zoster [shingles] affecting more than 50% of those aged 10–44 years at the introduction of vaccination."

Vaccine advocates point to studies that show no increase in shingles among those vaccinated. All cases that have had chicken pox have been mild. But since both the VZV and vaccine virus may remain dormant for many years, it will be decades before the answer is in. Will the vaccine virus be too weak to become activated? Or will the immunity induced by the vaccine be too weak to contain the virus?

CONCLUSION

Chicken pox vaccine is a live virus vaccine that is safe and effective in prevention of chicken pox in children. The unanswered questions about duration of immunity, the effect of shifting the age of infection upward, and the unknown effect on the occurrence of shingles in decades to come make universal vaccination of at best marginal benefit.[9] Given the present government policy of universal childhood vaccination, however, it may be unwise to try to avoid vaccination because of the hazard of later acquiring varicella as an adult.

CHAPTER 7

Diphtheria Vaccine

Ulcers occur on the tonsils, some mild and innocuous; but others pestilential, and fatal. . . . Such as are broad, hollow, foul and covered with black concretion, are pestilential. . . . If the disease extends to the tongue, the gums, and the alveoli and the teeth also become loosened and black; and the inflammation seizes the neck; and these die within a few days from the inflammation, fever, fetid smell and want of food.

THE ILLNESS

The above vivid description of what is probably diphtheria was written by Aretaeus the Cappadocian, whose practice flourished in Alexandria during the second century. He was renowned for his clinical skills and for revival of the by then five-hundred-year-old teachings of Hippocrates.[1] In the sixth century, Aaeius of Amida was known as a great Byzantine writer and physician to Emperor Justinian. He is quite an interesting character who apparently never had any formal medical training, and his famous sixteen-volume *Tetrabiblion* is mostly copied from the works of Galen and others. In addition to his writings on the use of pomegranate suppositories for contraception and the medicinal uses of wine, he did make some original and detailed studies of diphtheria.

A study of the disease, which was epidemic in the 1820s, was made by Pierre-Fidele Bretonneau, an epidemiologist trained during the French Revolution. He named the disease diphtheria from the Greek word for membrane, because of the membrane that forms in the throat. Bretonneau also performed the first successful tracheotomy, on a dining room table, in 1825.

A typical case of diphtheria starts out gradually after exposure to an infected individual. After one to five days, the child begins to feel sick. At first there are just a few patches in the throat, but if untreated these begin to coalesce and form the typical membrane. Although the child appears very ill, the temperature is only mildly increased. The glands in the side of the neck become greatly enlarged, causing the so-called bull neck appearance. If there are no complications, in about two weeks the membrane sloughs, sometimes in one whole cast of the throat and palate, and convalescence begins.

One of the most dangerous complications is blockage of the airways by the membrane. In such cases, tracheotomy may be lifesaving. It is necessary therefore to closely examine the patient's throat, but because of the pain, the child may refuse to be examined.[2]

Heart failure, a rapid and irregular pulse, and falling blood pressure are signs of heart muscle inflammation that sometimes occurs between the third and seventh days. It is usually fatal.

Neuropathy[3] is another potentially lethal complication, occurring in 20 percent of untreated patients. It begins two weeks to two months after the onset of the illness. The main symptom is muscular weakness such that the child cannot walk or use the arms. If the nerves about the head and neck are affected, the child may have difficulty swallowing or even breathing.

The overall mortality after infection is about 5 percent; it is higher in the very young and in older individuals. It should be noted, however, that the majority of children have only a mild illness or even no symptoms at all.

CORYNEBACTERIUM DIPHTHERIAE

Corynebacterium diphtheriae is the bacterium that causes diphtheria. It was first isolated and grown from a sample from the throat of a patient who had diphtheria in the 1880s. During the course of experimentation with the new "bug," investigators discovered that the soup in which the bacteria was cultured, when injected into hamsters, caused diphtheria. This was true even if the injected material contained no bacteria. It was apparent that Corynebacterium diphtheriae did not cause illness by invading the host, but by producing a powerful toxin. Three strains of Corynebacterium diphtheriae were identified: mitis, intermideus, and gravis, each more toxic than the last.

It was not until the twentieth century that scientists discovered how Corynebacterium diphtheriae makes the toxin. Researchers discovered the existence of bacteriophages, which are viruses that infect bacteria. It did not take long to find that Corynebacterium diphtheriae was infected with such a bacteriophage. The more dramatic discovery was that those strains of Corynebacterium diphtheriae that had no phage produced no toxin and so were harmless. It turns out that it is the bacteriophage that produces the toxin. Even more intriguing was the discovery that the bacteria control the phage and can switch the production of the toxin on or off. It is still not clear under what circumstances the switch is on or off, except that it is known that low iron concentration is needed for the switch to be on.

These observations explain some of the otherwise puzzling features of diphtheria, such as the unpredictable epidemics, and the presence of Corynebacterium diphtheriae in the community in the absence of diphtheria. An epidemic may occur in such a population if an outside phage invades the Corynebacterium diphtheriae or if the Corynebacterium diphtheriae decides to turn on a preexisting phage.

AÑO DE LOS GARROTILLOS

In Spain, 1613 was the year of *el garrotillos*, the strangler, when murderous diphtheria epidemics swept through Italy, Spain, and France. During the next century, epidemics erupted throughout Europe at roughly twelve-year intervals. The epidemiology of diphtheria is a study of the interaction of science, Corynebacterium diphtheriae, politics, war, and culture.

Diphtheria arrived in the American colonies in the eighteenth century, reaching epidemic proportions about 1735. Often whole families died in a few weeks. In the United States diphtheria is now virtually nonexistent. However, as late as 1890 some communities had 196 cases per 100,000 population, with 130 fatalities. Preschool and school-age children were mostly affected, but infants less than six months old appeared to be protected by maternal antibodies. Harry Truman developed diphtheria in 1894 when he was ten years old. He was paralyzed for months and had to be wheeled about in a baby carriage. Antitoxin was not then available, so he was treated with ipecac and whiskey. He developed a severe distaste for both.

Beginning in 1900, diphtheria deaths showed a dramatic, progressive drop to as low as fifteen per 100,000. This was before the diphtheria vaccines of the 1940s. The decrease in deaths may have been in part due to better treatment, including tracheotomy and antitoxin, but other common infectious diseases showed a similar, unexplained decrease.

In spite of the vaccine, there have been epidemics of diphtheria. During World War II, the invasion and disruption of the countries of Europe triggered an epidemic that became a pandemic, with over a million cases worldwide. Norwegian sailors brought diphtheria to Halifax, Nova Scotia, in 1940–41, causing an epidemic affecting 1 percent of the entire population. In 1943 an outbreak occurred in a German POW camp in Alabama.

Although there has been no major epidemic in the U.S. since 1890 and diphtheria is now rare in the U.S., pockets of diphtheria (known in the past as one of the "filth diseases") persist in scattered areas, especially in crowded or impoverished communities such as the Navajo reservation in Arizona and New Mexico, skid row in Seattle, the homes of aborigines of central Australia, and Inuit communities in Canada.

In the 1990s a major epidemic engulfed the newly independent states of the former Soviet Union. Diphtheria had been well controlled there for almost fifty years after universal childhood immunization was initiated in the 1950s. In 1976 there were only 198 cases. In the 1980s the immunization schedule was changed such that fewer doses of a possibly weaker vaccine were administered. Additionally, a powerful antivaccination movement arose associated with widespread distrust of the government during *perestroika* (1985–91). Alarmingly, in 1990 there was a 70 percent increase over the year before, presaging the explosion that followed in 1993. The subsequent epidemic had a toll of 140,000 cases and 4,000 deaths. A truly massive control program was initiated. Workers were vaccinated on the job, children in school, and others were vaccinated house-to-house. By 1995 the epidemic appeared to be contained and cases began to decrease.

The epidemic was caused by a number of factors. Most important was the development of a large population of adults who were susceptible, ironically because of childhood vaccination that had waned with time. Additionally, as noted above, the vaccination rate of children had fallen off considerably, creating many susceptible in that group as well. Other factors favoring the development of the epidemic were poverty, crowding, a large military population that was not immunized, and increased travel and population movement during those turbulent times.

Universal childhood vaccination and adult boosters would have prevented the epidemic.

THE VACCINE

In 1885, Kitasato Shibasaburo, a Japanese-trained physician and experimental bacteriologist, was invited to join the Institute of Hygiene in Berlin, headed by the legendary Robert Koch, who had assembled an enormously creative and productive group of researchers. It was the golden age of bacteriology. Among this group was Emil Adolph Behring, a Prussian-born bacteriologist. He and Kitasato teamed up to study the diphtheria toxin. In the course of their experiments, they found that if the toxin was heated before being injected, the guinea pig would live and, more important, it would then be immune to the effects of full-strength toxin. They theorized that the heated toxin had induced a substance in the guinea pig serum that could inactivate the diphtheria toxin. They named this substance antitoxin. They were in effect vaccinating the guinea pigs with the altered toxin. This altered toxin was far too potent to use in humans, but the antitoxin antibodies produced by guinea pigs and other animals could be used to treat rather than prevent diphtheria.[4]

The story goes that on Christmas night in 1891 in a Berlin clinic, a little girl lay dying of diphtheria. Behring injected her with the antitoxin. Her swift recovery seemed a miracle, and the era of "serum therapy" was born.

Kitasato returned to a prestigious and productive career in Japan the following year, but Behring became famous and wealthy and won the first Nobel Prize in medicine.[5] Within two years, antitoxin was being commercially manufactured in Germany in a firm founded by Behring. The firm, Aventis Behring, continues to manufacture biological serums to this day.

The advent of antitoxin therapy was greeted with enthusiasm worldwide. Victor Clarence Vaughan, in his charming 1926 autobiography, describes a medical meeting in 1894:

> In 1894 Doctor Novy and I attended the International Congress on Hygiene at Budapest and heard Roux read his paper on diphtheria antitoxin. This was given in an unventilated classroom of the musty old university. There were present many of the great men in preventive medicine from various parts of the world. At the conclusion of the reading these men stood on their seats, shouted applause in all civilized tongues and threw their hats toward the ceiling. I have never before nor since seen such a demonstration at a scientific congress. Each delegate returned to his home with a bottle of this marvelous curative agent in his possession.

In 1925 the town of Nome, Alaska, saw the onset of an epidemic of diphtheria. There was only a limited supply of antitoxin in the town, which could be reached only by dogsleds over 674 miles of ice and snow. Relays of dogs and men were urgently organized to get more antitoxin to Nome, and in less than two weeks the journey was completed, in time to save the town. There were twenty mushers, including Russians, Norwegians, Irish, and Indians. For the most part their names are forgotten, but

Balto, the lead dog of the last relay, is famous. There is a statue of him in Central Park in Manhattan, and he was the subject of a (very bad) movie. For the last thirty years the race to save Nome has been commemorated by the annual Iditarod dogsled race.

Of course, all was not romance. The serum was derived first from sheep, later horses. Administration of horse proteins sometimes causes serum sickness. The patient develops rash, fever, swollen joints, and swollen glands.

As described in a previous chapter, there was a disaster in St. Louis in 1901. The horse serum used for one particular batch of diphtheria antitoxin was contaminated with tetanus spores. This antiserum was given to twenty children, fourteen of whom died. The subsequent investigation showed that appropriate precautions in the preparation of the serum had been omitted. The fallout of the disaster led to the establishment of the predecessor of the Food and Drug Administration, the Biologics Control Act. Following the discovery of a preventive vaccine, antiserum usage was abandoned and now is available only from the CDC for treatment of the rare diphtheria infection.

Although the antiserum was highly effective in treating diphtheria cases, the search continued for a vaccine to prevent the disease. Von Behring found that in a mixture of toxin plus antitoxin, the toxin was neutralized but the mixture would still be able to induce a protective antibody. This preparation, TAM (toxin-antitoxin mixture), was 85 percent protective and relatively safe if the proportions of toxin and antitoxin were just right. Unfortunately this was not always the case. In 1919 in Dallas, a bad batch of TAM was given to three hundred children, with disastrous results (see the disaster chapter). Additionally, problems with horse serum continued. Better vaccines were discovered, and TAM passed into history in the 1920s.

So we arrive at the present-day diphtheria vaccine. In 1923, Alexander Glenny and Barbara Hopkins, working with diphtheria toxin in the United Kingdom, found that some of their samples had no toxin activity. They traced the source of the trouble to poor dishwashing technique; the glassware was contaminated with traces of formaldehyde, which totally neutralized the toxin. This was followed up by Gaston Ramon, a French veterinarian who preferred laboratory work to dealing with sick animals. Perhaps that was because as a young man during World War I he was assigned to produce antiserum by inoculating thousands of horses. In any case, his commanding officer, an infectious disease specialist, introduced Ramon to Emil Roux, director of the Pasteur Institute. Roux took Ramon on to work with the diphtheria vaccine. Like Glenny and Hopkins, Ramon found that formalin neutralizes the diphtheria toxin. He took the next giant step, which was to inoculate animals; they developed strong anti-body responses and were highly immune to diphtheria. The term toxoid was coined to indicate the modified toxin. The toxoid quickly replaced TAM because there was no active toxin in the preparation, and the horse serum problem was eliminated; the toxoid was a product of a laboratory. Nonetheless, there was opposition to the new vaccine; one reason cited was that the vaccine had been discovered by a veterinarian!

The present-day vaccine is prepared from cultures of Corynebacterium diphtheriae; the toxin-rich soup is purified, sterilized, and treated with formalin to produce the toxoid. Spoilage is prevented by adding thimerosal. Aluminum is added to enhance the efficacy of the toxoid. In the United States, diphtheria vaccine is available only combined with tetanus or tetanus-plus-pertussis vaccines.

Where the toxoid has been used extensively, diphtheria has been virtually eliminated. Some European countries have not had a single case in twenty years. Of concern, however, is the waning of immunity with time. Anti-body surveys show that as many as 50 percent of adults in some industrialized countries are susceptible. This creates the fertile ground for a possible breakout of diphtheria. Boosters for adults should therefore be routine.

Untoward reactions were very common in the early days of the toxoid. Recipients had severe reactions at the injection site and often fever and incapacitation for work for several days. Manufacturers of the vaccine purified the toxoid to remove contaminating bacterial products and reduced the dose considerably. Protection was just as good and side effects less. Still, reactions occurred, and were generally worse in adults and those partly immunized. Further advances came with the addition of aluminum salts that increased the potency of the toxoid, thus allowing an even smaller dose. The modern evaluation of adverse effects is clouded because the diphtheria toxoid is usually given with tetanus toxoid. Documented toxicity appears to be limited to local reactions and fever without serious complications.[6]

Immunization against diphtheria has a rocky history, but the modern vaccines are highly effective when used appropriately, with boosters, and have the potential of reducing clinical diphtheria to a rarity and maybe even someday eradicating this horrible disease.

CHAPTER 8

Pertussis (Whooping Cough) Vaccine

The whooping cough vaccines have been problematic from the start and, in spite of many advances, still are. There are at least eleven different kinds, none of which approaches 100 percent effectiveness, and all of which are associated with disturbing side effects. Even widespread immunization has not prevented an increase in whooping cough cases in the last twenty years. We delve into some bacteriology, immunology, and epidemiology to understand why this is so.

THE ILLNESS

Whooping cough typically goes through three phases. The first is the catarrhal phase, in which the child has what appears to be an ordinary cold. But instead of getting better, a cough starts in seven to fourteen days. A mild cough signals the onset of the second stage, the paroxysmal stage. The patient begins to have uncontrollable coughing fits, which end with a violent inhalation causing the "whoop." The attacks occur more frequently at night and may occur hourly or even more frequently. The child may appear well for a while until the next attack. As the disease progresses, the attacks become more frequent and violent. The child cannot breathe during the paroxysms and turns blue. The attack often terminates with vomiting and choking. This stage usually lasts two to four weeks, after which the cough continues but the whoop disappears, as the third, convalescent phase, begins. The cough gradually diminishes but may last weeks, even months.

Pneumonia, occurring in 5 percent of cases, is the most common fatal complication. Although whooping cough does not itself cause pneumonia, it paves the way for invasion by other pathogens.

Convulsions and brain damage causing permanent mental or neurologic deficits may be caused by the bacterial toxins or by the lack of oxygen during the cough spasms. Sometimes the cough is so violent that the lungs burst, ribs crack, eyes bleed, cerebral hemorrhage occurs, and hernias and rectum prolapse.

If the illness lasts longer than usual, starvation may occur because of all the vomiting. Evidence of starvation is obviously a bad sign and is particularly likely if the child was malnourished before the whooping cough started.

A strange feature of this strange disease is that whooping cough is much more common among female infants compared to male infants.

The older the patient, the milder the symptoms, contrary to the usual situation in which childhood diseases are more severe in adults. Infants under six months have the highest mortality.

In adults there may be no symptoms, or there may be simply a persisting cough, so the diagnosis depends on a positive culture or blood test. Such infected adults who have few or no symptoms commonly infect children in the household.

THE "BUG"

Whooping cough is caused by a very smart bacterium, Bordetella pertussis. There are two similar bacteria that cause a respiratory illness in domestic animals. The curious absence of clear-cut whooping cough before the sixteenth century suggests that the B. pertussis jumped from animal to man a mere five hundred years ago. This is conjectural, especially because some medical historians believe that the ancient folklore of southern India and Malabar do describe a whooping cough–like illness. If B. pertussis did jump from animals to man, it joins the company of other infections, including HIV (monkeys), tuberculosis (cows), influenza (pigs and ducks), and smallpox (cows).

Bordetella pertussis was named after its discoverer, the Nobel Prize–winner Jules-Jean-Baptiste-Vincent Bordet, who isolated the bacterium in 1906 at the Pasteur Institute in Brussels. His later, greater fame came from his work on immunity factors in blood serum.

B. pertussis produces several substances that cause the symptoms of whooping cough and depress the immune system of the patient. Three of these are particularly important, especially since they are the targets of the whooping cough vaccines. The first, FHA, glues the bacteria to the cells in the bronchial tubes. The second is pertussis toxin (PT), which is highly toxic to these cells and also depresses the host's immune system by blocking the attack of the white blood cells. The third is FIMS, which attacks the cells that have the microscopic cilia that brush foreign matter out of the respiratory tract. The combination of these and other elements cause the destruction of the lining of the bronchial tubes.

HISTORY

Whooping cough, commonly known in the late seventeenth century as chincough, was known to be infectious and contagious, but medical experts disagreed about almost everything else concerning it. Some argued that the symptoms arose from the chest, other argued in favor of the stomach or intestinal tract. These debates were made moot by an extraordinary Scotsman, Robert Watt. The youngest of three sons of a poor farmer, Robert had to work in the fields at an early age, and in his youth he toiled as a plowman and laborer in various locations in Scotland. During the course of his travels, he stayed briefly in the temporarily vacant home of Robert Burns. Excited by all the books there, Robert began a program of self-education, which secured him a place in Glasgow College, and later he received a doctorate in medicine from the University of Aberdeen.

This poor son of a poor farmer soon had a lucrative, even opulent, practice and was sought after as personal physician and teacher. But success did not save him from the grief of the loss to whooping cough of the two oldest of his four children. After their death he made a study of the disease, which culminated in the 1813 publication *Treatise on the History, Nature, and Treatment of Chincough*. His meticulous dissections laid the foundation for the modern understanding of this disease.

VACCINES

The earliest vaccines were crude suspensions of formalin-killed B. pertussis cultures. Since whole bacteria were used, all the elements produced by the bacteria, known and unknown, were included in these "whole cell" vaccines. First licensed in the USA in 1914, they were often contaminated with other bacteria and varied in potency from lot to lot and manufacturer to manufacturer. Some lots were effective in producing antibodies and others showed no effect at all. Almost all contain aluminum salts, which boosts the vaccine's potency, as well as mercury as a preservative. The four whole-cell vaccines available in the U.S. today are made by Connaught, Wyeth-Lederle, and the Massachusetts and Michigan public health departments. When these are compared, there are large differences in the antibody response to the various components of the vaccines. The clinical importance of these variations is unknown, since they were never compared head-to-head. A further complication is that the overall response to the whole-cell vaccine depends in part on the level of maternal antibodies. These antibodies usually disappear by age four months.[1] Since 1948 the whole-cell vaccine has been administered combined with tetanus and diphtheria toxoid (DPT).

In 1981, Japanese scientists were able to extract PT, FIMS, and FHA from the whole cell. Vaccines against these purified antigens were soon to follow. Since these purified vaccines no longer contained the whole bacterial cell, they were dubbed "acellular" and notated as "aP," as in DaPT. The hope, only partially realized, was that the acellular vaccines would be effective and have fewer side effects than the whole-cell vaccines.

Today the acellular vaccines are made by at least eleven different manufacturers, each with different amounts of some or all of the three antigens. Instead of mercury, the preservative is phenoxyethanol. Although the inexpensive whole-cell vaccines continue in worldwide use, it is likely that they will disappear from the U.S. marketplace in the next few years.

EFFICACY

The efficacy of the various whooping cough vaccines has been studied, analyzed, hotly debated, proclaimed, and denied for almost ninety years.

The first large-scale trial of whooping cough vaccine was conducted in the Faeroe Islands. This tiny country of eighteen rocky islands sits in the North Atlantic Ocean, halfway between Norway and Iceland. Almost all the inhabitants are descendants of the Vikings who settled there in the eighth century. Epidemics of whooping cough occurred there in 1924 and 1929. A whole-cell vaccine was used in an attempt to halt the epidemics. It is not clear how effective it was, but there was some degree of protection, and vaccinated persons who did become infected had milder cases. Because the diagnosis depended on symptoms alone, many patients may have been misclassified. During the second epidemic, however, one event, which has haunted the whooping cough vaccine ever since, was unquestioned: two children died. Both had received the vaccine within a week of birth. One had convulsions before death.

Efficacy studies prior to the 1940s depended on clinical trials because available blood tests for antibody levels did not correlate with efficacy.

These early clinical trials had all the usual problems of carrying out large-scale population studies, made more difficult by the variety of vaccines produced by various manufacturers, no two of which were alike. Predictably, some studies showed a high degree of protection and some showed virtually none.

The first useful laboratory test for evaluating whooping cough vaccines was the "mouse protection" test. The mouse was immunized with the vaccine, and then live B. pertussis bacteria was injected into the brain. Gruesome as this test may be, it did allow for some degree of standardization of the many vaccines being studied. The mouse protection test, still required by the FDA, has been the standard laboratory test for vaccine potency for over forty years. Only recently has it been found that some inactive vaccines can pass the test.

According to K.M. Edwards et al. in Plotkin, "Although studies with early vaccines produced inconsistent results, clinical trials subsequent to the standardization of the vaccines by the mouse protection test demonstrated clear-cut, consistent efficacy." But she cites only three papers. One is a 1936 immunization progress report[2] that predates the mouse protection test, the second is a 1947 report in the *Journal of Pediatrics*,[3] and the last is a 1959 report to the British Immunization Council.[4]

In attempts to further study efficacy, nine clinical trials were conducted between 1985 and 1993. All of these trials used acellular vaccine; some also included whole-cell vaccine. The Swedish efficacy trial in 1986 compared two different acellular vaccines with placebo in a study of 3,800 children. Although it was a double-blind, well-designed study, interpretation of the results depended heavily on the criteria used to diagnose whooping cough. Counting all cough illnesses gives the vaccine a very poor efficacy rate, but counting only prolonged cough cases with a positive culture would show very high efficacy. It was a two-dose study, at five to eleven months and eight to twelve weeks later. The efficacy of the better of the two was judged to be only 69 percent. These vaccines were withdrawn because of the poor efficacy and concern about the possibility of a unique toxicity. Four children died of overwhelming bacterial infection: Two had meningitis, one had pneumonia, the other blood poisoning. This suggested that the vaccines may have impaired the children's immunity. A cause and effect was never established.

Another Swedish study (Stockholm, 1993) compared two acellular vaccines with a whole-cell vaccine and a placebo. These were randomized, double-blinded studies. The acellular vaccines were 59 percent to 85 percent effective; the whole-cell vaccine was only 48 percent effective.

Yet another Swedish study in Goteborg had an efficacy estimated at 54 to 77 percent. This was an acellular vaccine containing only the antitoxin antigen.

A trial in Munich, Germany, in 1993–95 reported 93–96 percent efficacy of both an acellular and a whole-cell vaccine. This unfortunately was an unblinded, nonrandomized study, the design of which could cause a serious overestimation of efficacy.

Another German trial was conducted in Erlangen from 1991–94. The vaccines studied were a cellular and an acellular vaccine. The acellular vaccine had an efficacy of 78 percent; the whole-cell 93 percent. But once again the devil was in the details of the trial design. This study was conducted in the private offices of local physicians. Depending on how hard they looked for cases, efficacy estimates varied from 40 to 75 percent.[5]

Niakhar, Senegal, was the site of a clinical trial from 1990 to 1994. This study compared a whole-cell vaccine, an acellular vaccine, a DT (diphtheria-tetanus combination), and no vaccine. The whole-cell vaccine had a 92 percent efficacy compared to the acellular vaccine at 74 percent. This study aroused some controversy and criticism because of the small number of subjects (less than 500) and other problems in the study design.

There are other measures of vaccine efficacy besides clinical trials. Although antibody levels do not correlate well with vaccine efficacy, they are of value in comparing one vaccine with another and estimating the duration of immunity. In some cases antibody levels after vaccination are higher than after natural infection, but they are frequently lower and decline much faster.

EPIDEMIOLOGY

Demographic data show that there has been a dramatic decline in whooping cough in developed countries. But like some other illnesses, such as rheumatic fever and tuberculosis, whooping cough began mysteriously declining before the vaccine era. This phenomenon is usually attributed to better nourishment and "improved social and economic conditions." In spite of the spontaneous decline, a close look at demographic data show that with the advent of whooping cough vaccine, there was a further decline to the point of virtual eradication in some areas that had a high vaccination rate. In 1976 in the U.S., there were only 1,010 cases reported, a 99 percent drop from the prevaccination era. In subsequent years, however, the number of cases began to increase, reaching a peak of over 7,000 in 1996. There have been cyclical peaks in the number of cases in three-to-four-year cycles; each peak has been higher than the one before. We may well be simply on the downside of the present cycle, in which case there will be a further rise. In 1993, after twenty years of a stable, low rate of infection, an epidemic of pertussis affecting 352 persons occurred in Cincinnati. There was a dramatic shift in the age distribution of patients from infants toward older immunized children, adolescents, and adults. Most disturbing was the occurrence of epidemic pertussis among children who were appropriately immunized for their age. Eighty-five percent of the children six to twelve years old who had pertussis had received four or more doses of the DPT vaccine. The authors of the report of the epidemic very cautiously concluded that "since the 1993 pertussis epidemic in Cincinnati occurred primarily among children who had been appropriately immunized, it is clear that the whole-cell pertussis vaccine failed to give full protection against the disease."[6] It should be noted, however, that most of the cases were mild and there were no deaths. There was a similar epidemic in Chicago in 1993.

The cause of this disturbing increase of cases is unknown. Waning immunity may be the explanation. This fits with the observation that the increase in cases has occurred predominantly among adolescents and adults. Some studies have shown that vaccination with three or fewer doses is associated with early loss of protection (but this did not apply to the Cincinnati epidemic). At best, vaccine-induced immunity starts to decline four years after the last dose. The obvious "fix" would be to give boosters to older children and adults. But because of increased side effects, no whooping cough vaccine has been licensed for this group, in whom whooping cough complications are rare. However, because of the finding that adults are a reservoir of B. pertussis, there has been renewed interest in a vaccine for adults. Several acellular vaccines are currently being tested.

Another possible cause of the increasing number of cases is a change in the bacteria or in the vaccine. So far, however, no such change has been detected.

Strong evidence of the benefits of pertussis vaccine was provided by unintended experiments that occurred in three developed countries when vaccine use was curtailed or abandoned.[7]

Hyakunichi-zeki, "the cough lasting one hundred days," known as pertussis in the West, was epidemic in postwar Japan. In 1949–50 there were reported 150 cases per 100,000 population. The true rate was probably ten times higher. In 1950, mandatory vaccination was instituted, and the case rate fell from 150 to 0.2 per 100,000. In 1975, two children died after receiving whole-cell whooping cough vaccine: one from shock and the other from brain damage. The vaccine was temporarily suspended and when resumed was administered only to children at least two years old. Nonetheless, vaccination rates fell dramatically. Soon whooping cough was again epidemic, peaking in 1979. In 1980, an effective acellular vaccine was introduced and cases decreased rapidly, with the majority occurring in under-two-year-old (unimmunized) children.

A virtual boycott of the vaccine in 1975 in England and Wales was followed by two major epidemics, in 1977–79 and 1982–83.[8]

Immunization with whole-cell vaccine was introduced in Sweden in 1950 but cases continued to appear, and the vaccine was discontinued in 1979. After the usual three-to-four-year lull, cases began to increase in number, reaching epidemic proportions in 1983 and 1985.

So, what are we to make of all this? Many questions remain, but it is most unlikely that additional clinical trials will provide answers. The effort and expense and lack of profit in attempting a trial large enough to give "definitive" data means that what information we have is all we will get. Looking over all the efficacy data, one can say that all the whooping cough vaccines now in common use are effective to one degree or another, probably in the 75 percent range. Nonetheless, because of herd immunity, an effective vaccination program can be associated with a near-zero incidence even though a sizable proportion of the population is susceptible.

It is unclear if the whole-cell vaccine is more or less effective than the various acellular vaccines, but the acellular vaccines are, as we shall see, less toxic.

TOXICITY

As we have already noted, side effects have bedeviled whooping cough vaccines from the outset. Plotkin notes, under the heading "Common reactions," local reactions, fever, and excesssive somnolence (drowsiness) in about half the children vaccinated. Some have an abnormally deep sleep that may last for a day. Others emit strange, high-pitched screams unlike any other; the screaming may go on for hours. Still others have incessant inconsolable weeping and crying.

Uncommon reactions (about 0.06 percent) include convulsions with fever. Another rare side effect is HHE (hypotonic-hyporesponsive episodes). It comes on suddenly, minutes to hours after immunization. The child becomes listless or unconscious and goes completely limp. The skin is very pale. The condition can last for a few minutes or as long as forty-eight hours. All recover.

We now come to the contentious and distressing subject of the brain damage known as encephalopathy. The child rapidly regresses and may become listless or lapse into total unconsciousness. Seizure, paralysis, and even death may follow. These symptoms may have many causes, so the question is whether or not the encephalopathy is due to the vaccine. To the parents who witness a well child becoming ill hours or days after vaccination, there is no doubt about the answer. They will consider no alternative. To the statistician, however, the case is not proven until there are statistically significant data showing cause and effect. In this instance such data is almost impossible to come by because there are so few cases that coincidence cannot be ruled out. To the public health official this issue is important but not decisive, because even if rare cases of encephalopathy are caused by the vaccine, the benefit of preventing whooping cough still far outweighs the risk. To family doctors, encephalopathy is to risk daily a misfortune that hopefully will not befall their young patients or themselves.

In 1994 the IOM (Institute of Medicine of the National Academy of Science), after exhaustive review of all the evidence, concluded that "the balance of evidence is consistent with a causal relation between DPT and chronic nervous system dysfunction in children whose serious acute neurologic illness occurred within 7 days of . . . vaccination." The best available guess is that encephalopathy occurs once in 310,000 doses.

There have been other, totally unsubstantiated allegations of whooping cough vaccine toxicity. In the early 1980s several reports linked sudden infant death syndrome (SIDS) to whooping cough vaccine. Subsequent comprehensive studies showed no causal relation. Autism, ADD, epilepsy, anemia, and diabetes have been attributed to whooping cough vaccination, but without any convincing evidence.

The acellular vaccines have been shown, in many studies, to have the same side effects as the traditional whole-cell vaccine, but at a much decreased rate, averaging two-thirds fewer side effects.

CONCLUSION

Whooping cough vaccine has prevented countless deaths; vaccination is an important public health benefit, but at the cost of frequent side effects and rare instances of encephalopathy. As late as 1977 a *Lancet* editorial questioned the risk/benefit ratio. The advent of the acellular vaccines will tip the balance toward the benefit side.

Wherever possible, acellular vaccines should be used. The vaccine is generally administered in combination with other vaccines, usually as DaTP, of which there are several different ones licensed for use in the U.S. In the absence of evidence that any one of them is superior to the others, the choice of vaccine will probably depend on price, availability, and the manufacturers' marketing strategy.

CHAPTER 9

Tetanus Vaccine

Tetanus is a grisly disease that, unlike most other vaccine-preventable diseases, is not passed from person to person. The bacterium that causes tetanus, Clostridium tetani, is present in the soil all over the world, and in cow dung, horse manure, human feces, and the intestines of many other animals. In its dormant (spore) stage it causes no illness. The spores are almost indestructible, tolerating heat, cold, chemicals, and drought. But when conditions are favorable, Clostridium tetani becomes active and produces a lethal poison (tetanospasmin) that ravages the nervous system. It is even more potent than the deadly diphtheria toxin. Tetanus spores become active only in the absence of oxygen, which is a poison to these bacteria.[1]

TETANUS OF THE NEWBORN

Tetanus of the newborn occurs through contamination of the umbilical stump (and occasionally as a complication of circumcision). Neonatal tetanus is common in some cultures that have practices that encourage infection. Some tribes in the Loralai district of Pakistan practice "bundling," in which the lower abdomen of the newborn is smeared with cow dung and then the child is wrapped in a sheepskin blanket. The Masai have a high neonatal death rate in part due to the custom of packing the umbilical stump with cow dung. In the Sudan the cord is tied with blades of grass, bark fibers, reeds, or fine roots that may be contaminated with Clostridium tetani spores. A variety of tools are used to cut the cord. They are usually items that are available in the house or that relate to the father's trade, such as scissors, knives, broken glass, stones, sickles, or used razor blades. These are rarely cleaned or boiled before use and are dangerous sources of infection. In some parts of India, ghee (clarified butter) is applied to the stump. This practice is associated with high infection rates in those communities that heat the ghee by burning cow dung.

In a typical case of neonatal tetanus, the newborn appears healthy and takes well to the breast, but in eight days (plus or minus four days) the baby becomes ill. The first symptoms are poor sucking and excessive crying. Facial muscle spasms interfere with sucking and swallowing. Spasm of the back muscles makes the infant rigid. If the infection is mild, recovery may begin after a week, but many of the children die.

Neonatal tetanus is common in developing countries but rare in the United States. Since 1984 there have been only two cases reported in the USA. Neonatal tetanus can be largely prevented by clean, antiseptic care of the umbilical stump. In the first half of the nineteenth century, on the small rocky island of Vestmannaeyjaar[2] in Iceland, over 60 percent of all children died before the age of one year. Most died in the first two weeks of life, usually of neonatal tetanus. A series of public health measures was followed by a dramatic drop in mortality. This was decades before the bacteriologic revolution found its way to Iceland. Similar, if less dramatic, decreases in neonatal tetanus occurred in developing countries when antiseptic (or at least clean) methods of umbilical care were instituted. Nonetheless, neonatal tetanus continues to be a problem in parts of the world where immunization is refused or unavailable.

Immunization against neonatal tetanus depends on immunization of the mother before or during pregnancy. The mother's antibodies protect the child for about six months. There is even some evidence that the fetus produces its own antibodies in response to the tetanus vaccine.[3]

Treatment of neonatal tetanus depends on maintaining adequate nourishment and fluids and the use of tetanus antitoxin, preferably of human origin.

TETANUS IN ADULTS

Tetanus in adults usually occurs as a complication of a wound or injury of an unimmunized individual. The classic case is a puncture wound of the foot due to a loose barn floor nail. This provides a large dose of Clostridium tetani spores (manure) and a low oxygen environment (the puncture), which is the perfect setting for tetanus. Other at-risk penetrating injuries include bullet wounds, industrial injuries, self-performed body piercing, tattooing, animal bites, and intravenous drug use. In 1997, of eleven reported cases of tetanus in California, six occurred among intravenous drug (especially heroin) users. Abrasions, lacerations, open fractures, and abscesses may also lead to tetanus. At least three cases have occurred following surgery. Sometimes even an apparently minor wound, not even noticed, may result in tetanus.

Symptoms usually start in a few days, but may be delayed for weeks. The first symptom is spasm of the chewing muscles, giving rise to the name lockjaw. As the spasms increase, the patient's face is distorted into a gruesome grin (risus sardonicus). The spasms spread to all the muscles and are so intense that the victims may break their bones or injure their spine. The reflexes become so hyperactive that even a loud noise can throw the entire body into agonizing rigidity. Spasm of the throat muscles can cause instant death. Complications include heart and circulatory failure, pneumonia, blood clots, and bedsores.[4] Ellen Bolte has proposed that low-grade chronic tetanus infection may contribute to the occurrence of autism. Mortality depends on the location of the injury, the degree of contamination, availability of tetanus antitoxin, and access, when necessary, to intensive care, including intravenous muscle relaxers and respirators.

Tetanus in adults occurs almost exclusively in persons who are not adequately immunized. It can be prevented to a limited extent by good wound care, especially the removal of the dead tissue that favors Clostridium tetani growth. Further treatment depends on the person's immunization history. Unless the wound is at high risk, no additional immunization is needed if the patient has had a three-dose primary vaccination and a booster within five years. If more than five years, a booster should be given. Depending on the wound, tetanus antitoxin (see below) may also be administered. If the individual has not had a full primary tetanus toxoid series, they should be given both the toxoid (for long-term protection) and antitoxin (TIG) for immediate protection.

TETANUS ANTITOXIN

In 1889, Kitasato Shibasaburo, working in Robert Koch's laboratory in Berlin, was able to isolate and grow Clostridium tetani in pure culture. This made possible the identification of tetanus toxin. Antitoxin, consisting of antibodies against the toxin, was developed soon after. As in the case of diphtheria, the antitoxin antibodies were induced by injecting horses with the toxin and then harvesting their serum. The antitoxin provides passive immunity in that it does not stimulate antibody formation but provides preformed antibodies. As a therapeutic or preventive agent, the horse serum has major shortcomings. Some persons had adverse reactions to the horse serum, which were sometimes serious and even fatal. Furthermore, the antitoxin lasts only about two weeks. Nonetheless, this was an important piece of medical armament, especially in the Great War. In all, 8.5 million soldiers died, more than half due to illness. In the muddy fields of Flanders and in the trenches of Verdun, tetanus-prone injuries were common. U.S. forces experienced fourteen cases of tetanus per 100,000 combatants. The antitoxin saved many lives. By 1960, however, the horse serum was replaced with the safer and more effective tetanus immune globulin (TIG).

TIG is human tetanus antitoxin. It is extracted from serum of persons who have a high level of antitoxin due to effective immunization or recovery from natural tetanus. The effect of TIG lasts for a month, twice as long as the horse serum.

The potential downside of TIG is that, since it is a mix of the plasma of hundreds of donors, exposure to any possible blood-borne infection is enormous. Even though each donor unit is verified to be negative for HIV and hepatitis, it is theoretically possible that other infections may survive the sterilization methods used. At present there is no screening for parvovirus or the Jakob-Kreutzfeld (human mad cow disease) agent or SV40 monkey virus.

There are many brands of TIG, all a little bit different. Tetramune is used in the USA.

TETANUS TOXOID

Tetanus toxoid is the agent used for routine immunization. It consists of tetanus toxoid that has been inactivated by formaldehyde so that it is harmless but still able to stimulate an antibody response. It became commercially available in 1938, but was not in widespread use until the early forties.

In 1942 two Germans, K. L. Wolters and H. Dehmal, immunized each other with their toxoid and then administered a lethal dose of tetanus antitoxin. Both survived.

A double-blind randomized control trial reported in 1966 showed that immunization of women of childbearing age in Colombia resulted in a dramatic drop in neonatal tetanus. The control group experienced seventy-eight cases per 1,000 live births; the immunized group had no cases.

In World War II there were 2.7 million U.S. servicemen wounded; only four cases of tetanus occurred in those who had been immunized.

Immunity wanes in time, and so booster shots are given in adolescence and every ten years thereafter.

The toxoid is prepared by growing Clostridium tetani in huge vats. The soup has no animal products but contains aluminum, formaldehyde, and thimerosal. The potency of the toxoid is measured by how well it protects guinea pigs from an otherwise lethal dose of tetanus toxin.

Local reactions such as pain, swelling, and redness at the injection site are common. Their severity depends in part on the potency of the preparation, the way it is injected, the aluminum content; reactions tend to be more severe with each subsequent dose. Many manufacturers produce many variations of the toxoid. The side effect picture is clouded by the routine use of DPT or other combinations with the tetanus toxoid.

Rare but serious side effects are damage to the nerves in the arm and shoulder and, possibly, even the spinal cord. And, as is the case with almost any vaccine or medication, an immediate, life-threatening anaphylactic shock can occur.

CONCLUSION

Tetanus toxoid is one of the most effective and safest of vaccines. Since exposure to the spores is unavoidable, and since herd immunity does not exist, all individuals, in the absence of known allergy to the toxoid, should be fully immunized.

CHAPTER 10

Measles Vaccine

Measles was first described in the seventh century by the famous Hebrew physician, Al Yehudi. It appears that he included cases that were other types of illnesses as well. Three hundred years later, the Persian Rhazes distinguished measles from other rashes, including smallpox. The first attempts to prevent measles through immunization were made in the mid-eighteenth century when a Scottish physician, Francis Home, inoculated twelve children with material from the blood of a measles patient. Ten of the children developed a mild measles infection. The technique, known as morbillisation, was never widely adopted. It was not until the mid-twentieth century that measles immunization became established.

THE ILLNESS

Measles is caused by the measles virus and is one of the most contagious of illnesses. The patient is infective for three to four days before the rash appears, and as it fades, so does the infectivity. A typical case in the industrialized world starts with a cough, fever, weakness, and malaise. On about the fourth day, the rash appears. It begins on the face and spreads out to the trunk, arms, and legs. It starts out as spots, but the spots may merge to cause an overall redness. The rash fades away and the patient recovers completely in a few days. Complications include pneumonia in 1 to 6 percent, ear infections that can cause deafness in 7 to 9 percent (Plotkin), and rare infection of the eyes can cause blindness. Diarrhea is common and may be long-lasting and life-threatening.

The most devastating potential complication is SSPE (subacute sclerosing panencephalitis). It usually occurs seven years after measles infection and gradually destroys the brain. Intellect suffers first, followed by personality changes, seizures, paralysis, and death. Mercifully, this is rare, occurring in one per 100,000 cases.

These complication rates are a low percentage, but since all children become infected in the absence of the vaccine, the number of affected children is in the hundreds of thousands. In my opinion this warrants widespread administration of measles vaccine. The need for the vaccine is much greater in Third World countries, where measles has a much more ugly face. Perhaps because of malnutrition and vitamin A deficiency, measles carries 5 to 15 percent mortality, usually due to pneumonia or dehydration due to diarrhea. Before they die, the children sometimes bleed under the skin; this is called "black measles."

The measles vaccine contains an attenuated, weakened measles virus that induces immunity to measles but does not cause measles itself. The measles virus is made relatively harmless by passing it through various animal tissues. There are at least eleven different varieties of measles vaccine, each with its own slightly different strain. In Asia, a strain grown in dog cells is used. In the United States, the Moraton strain is used. This measles virus, isolated from Master Edmonston in the mid-1900s, was attenuated by serial passage through human kidney cells, human amniotic fluid, and chick embryo cells. The vaccine so prepared had frequent side effects, so it was further attenuated by passage through chicken cells or human cell cultures. It is usually administered in combination with mumps and rubella vaccines (MMR). Unlike the other live vaccine viruses, polio and smallpox, the measles vaccine virus is not transmittable from person to person.

A formalin-inactivated killed vaccine was licensed in 1963. This vaccine was not only ineffective but also sometimes made subsequent measles worse. It caused an atypical rash, which starts out in the arms and legs and moves to the trunk and head; this is the reverse of the natural infection. It was abandoned in 1967, by which time 1.8 million doses had been administered. There is no detailed information about this episode in the mainstream medical literature.

The currently used live vaccine is highly effective. When administered in an appropriate setting, the vaccine has reduced measles cases to near zero. The vaccine is so effective that if enough resources are available, global measles eradication is possible within a decade.

The timing of the first dose of routine measles vaccination has been problematic. Since the younger the infant, the worse the measles, immunization should be given at the earliest possible age. However, the newborn has maternal measles antibodies that prevent the vaccine from working—these antibodies dissipate in time. When first licensed in 1963, it was recommended that the first dose be given at age nine months. It was found, however, that many infants still had antibodies from the mother, so in 1965 the age was increased to twelve months. In subsequent years, it was found that children vaccinated at age twelve months lost their immunity sooner than older children did, so in 1976 the age was changed to fifteen months. In 1994 the age was yet again changed to twelve months because the mothers, having been immunized with the measles vaccine in childhood, had lower antibodies levels than did the mothers in the prevaccine era.

Side effects are common. Up to 15 percent of children have fever after the first dose. It usually begins seven to twelve days after the inoculation. As with any other fever, some children have febrile convulsions. About 5 percent of children have a rash at seven to ten days. Reactions to subsequent doses are milder than the first except in the rare case of rash and joint pain, especially in older children.

A drop in blood platelets (thrombocytopenia) occurs in one per 30,000 cases, but this had not caused bleeding or other complications.

More problematic are the many individual reports of a variety of neurological complications, occurring in the magnitude of one case per million doses. These are so rare that it is impossible to know if the association between vaccine and neurological damage is side effect or coincidence.

Two children have died from overwhelming measles vaccine virus; both had severe immune system deficiency.

In its February 28, 1998, issue, *The Lancet* published an article that caused a storm of controversy that battered the scientific and medical worlds, the media, the government, public health services, and the population at large, especially parents of young children and parents of autistic children. Andrew Wakefield, the author, reported on eleven children who developed autism after receiving measles vaccine. Wakefield, a charismatic and flamboyant British surgeon, publicly called for a halt to measles vaccination. Subsequent studies by many different groups of specialists in many different countries have shown that measles vaccine has nothing to do with autism.

CHAPTER 11

Mumps Vaccine

The origin of the word mumps is lost in the haze of antiquity. In the fifth century, Hippocrates described in his *Book of Epidemics* what sounds like mumps. The modern study of the illness, however, begins with R. Hamilton in 1790. In a paper titled "An Account of a distemper by the common people of England vulgarly called the mumps,"[1] he was the first to recognize the neurological damage caused by mumps and described the inflammation of the testicles (orchitis).

Although mumps has been considered one of the "usual" childhood diseases, it has also occurred in epidemic form, especially in the military. In World War I, more than 200,000 servicemen were hospitalized with mumps, and it had the distinction of being second in diseases only to gonorrhea (and influenza). The last large military epidemic was aboard the SS *Reuben James* stationed in the eastern Pacific in 1992.

Mumps is caused by a virus that is transmitted by coughing, sneezing, or other contact with saliva. About two weeks after exposure, in the typical case, there is painful swelling of one or both parotid glands (the salivary glands in front of and below the ear, overlying the angle of the jaw). The patient has fever for as long as a week. In almost half the cases the only symptoms are those of a cold, and the diagnosis is usually missed. It is therefore common for persons to be unaware that they have had mumps.

Orchitis affects the testicles in adults much more often than in young children. It causes pain, embarrassment, and apprehension far more commonly than it causes sterility, which is rare, even if both testicles are involved. Another complication more common among adults is breast inflammation, occurring in about a third of infected women.

The most common complication of mumps is meningitis or encephalitis caused by virus in the brain. Complete recovery is the rule, although there are unfortunate exceptions. Mumps is the most common cause of acquired childhood deafness. It occurs in only one per 20,000 cases, but when mumps infection was almost universal, it added up to many cases.

The mumps virus affects numerous other organs including the heart, pancreas, kidneys, and joints, but these complications are rare.

The first mumps vaccine was a killed vaccine, approved for general use in the forties. But immunity was short-lived, and that vaccine was abandoned after live vaccines became available in the sixties. There are presently more than ten different live vaccine strains in use. All are attenuated mumps viruses, created by passage through various animal and human tissues. The mumps vaccine virus is grown in chick embryo cells in the presence of gelatin and neomycin antibiotic and so may cause allergic reactions in persons sensitive to those components of the vaccine.

There are differences in efficacy and toxicity among the strains, the most notable being the relatively high rate of meningitis following administration of the Urabe strain, which is still widely used in Japan and other countries because it produces high antibody levels.

The so-called Jeryl Lynn strain is used in the United States. It is actually a combination of two viral strains. It is usually administered in combination with measles and rubella vaccines in the MMR vaccine. Following licensure of the live vaccine, the number of reported mumps cases in the U.S. fell from 152,209 to an all-time low of 2,982 in 1985. As immunity wore off, there was a rise in cases in 1986 to 1989, but with the administration of the vaccine in multiple doses of MMR, mumps cases are now down to less than a thousand per year. Nonetheless, outbreaks have occurred in at least two high schools that had 95 percent vaccination rates. It is unclear if this is due to a waning of immunity or a primary failure of the vaccine to work in the first place. What is clear is that protection in the field is a lot lower than it is in controlled clinical trials, and the vaccine is not as protective as is the natural infection.

As we have seen in other cases, immunization of young children may cause a shift of infection into adulthood, when the disease is more severe. Administration of booster doses in adolescence is usually recommended to avoid this problem, which is due to a waning of the childhood immunization.

The most common side effect of the vaccine is an illness similar to a mild case of the mumps. Rarely, the vaccine causes symptoms like the complications of mumps itself: orchitis, arthritis, deafness, and muscle inflammation.

Many of the mumps vaccine viruses cause meningitis. The Jeryl Lynn strain causes meningitis in one in 800,000 doses, which is much lower than the number of cases that would occur naturally in the absence of vaccine. No permanent damage is done by the vaccine-induced meningitis. Twenty-six states have made mumps immunization mandatory, and those states have the fewest cases of mumps.

CHAPTER 12

Rubella Vaccine

The rubella story has elements of genius, tragedy, luck, and redemption. Rubella begins with a mild flulike illness, and a few days later a pink rash appears, starting on the face and spreading to the torso and limbs. Frequently there are swollen glands in the back of the neck and at the base of the skull. Sometimes there are no symptoms at all except for the rash, and in some cases even the rash is absent, but blood tests show that an infection has occurred. Therefore it is not unusual for someone to have had rubella and not know it. Some children and many adults have painful swollen joints for a few days. A rare complication is meningitis. In the vast majority of cases, the patient is well in a few days.

We have no idea where rubella came from, or when. It was "discovered" in the late eighteenth century, when it was first distinguished from the other rashes of the time. Because the first descriptions appeared in German medical journals, the illness became known as "German measles." Or perhaps German measles is a corruption of "germane" measles, germane in the sense of "closely akin to." Rubella was also known as the "three-day measles" because the rash usually subsides in three days. In any case, it was Henry Vale, a Scottish physician stationed in India, who described an outbreak in a boys' school and coined the term rubella. He liked that name "because it is short for the sake of convenience in writing and euphonious for ease in pronunciation."[1] For the ensuing one hundred years, rubella attracted little interest in medical circles, being considered a benign, minor illness.

In 1941, however, an Australian ophthalmologist, Sir Norman McAllister Gregg, was seeing a disturbingly large number of infants who had congenital cataracts. McAllister, then in his fiftieth year, was one of the few ophthalmologists in Sydney who was not in the military, so he saw many cases. One day he overheard the mothers of two of his patients comparing notes in the hallway. Both women had infants with cataracts, and both had had German measles while pregnant. Up until that time, although he was a highly trained and respected physician, McAllister's main claim to fame was his prowess on the tennis courts and in cricket. But the overheard conversation was all the stimulation McAllister needed to turn to his clinical data and make the discovery that rubella during pregnancy caused congenital cataracts. He could tell that these cataracts were unlike other congenital cataracts and that they had occurred when the fetus was a few weeks old. Virtually all the mothers of affected babies had had German measles in the first trimester. The large number of cases correlated with the Australian epidemic of rubella in the encampments surrounding Sydney.

In his original paper, McAllister noted that some of the children had other congenital anomalies, including heart disease. When he presented his findings to his Australian colleagues, he was praised for his discovery. McAllister later became a much-honored hero. But at first the wider medical community was very skeptical. As late as 1947, *The Lancet* declared that McAllister's hypothesis was "not proven."

Fast forward to 1951. As Professor Henry Oliver Lancaster, a brilliant and innovative mathematician and statistician, passes by the old Australian Institute for the Deaf and Dumb, he has an idea: Could the records in the institute have hidden in them a possible connection between rubella and deafness? It turns out that the old hospital had marvelously detailed records, as did the Australian health services. In a statistical tour de force, Lancaster demonstrated an almost absolute correlation between rubella cases and congenital deafness.

Soon reports of rubella-induced deformities of virtually all organs of the afflicted fetuses were coming in from all over the world—the term CRS (congenital rubella syndrome) was used to signify this whole spectrum of anomalies. There was little doubt that rubella in pregnancy caused fetal abnormalities and did so in 90 percent of early pregnancies.

Rubella is a worldwide infection. The age at infection varies from area to area. Typically, it affects the majority of children who live in close quarters. In circumstances in which there is no crowding and in which hygiene and nutrition are good, the age at infection is older. Young adults in schools, the military, and even the Wall Street stock market have been the patients of outbreaks. This upward shift of age has important implications, as we shall see.

In the United States, before the rubella vaccine, each spring brought a crop of cases. Superimposed on this periodicity were major epidemics at seven-year intervals. The last major U.S. epidemic was in 1964–65. The numbers tell what words cannot express: 12.5 million cases of rubella; 2,084 cases of encephalitis; 2,100 deaths at birth; 6,250 miscarriages; 8,055 deaf children; 3,580 deaf-blind children; 1,790 mentally retarded children; other abnormalities 6,575; therapeutic abortions 5,000.

There have been numerous other epidemics, including the Australian one in the forties, but none other was so well documented.

With this background, let us look at the rubella vaccine. The currently used rubella vaccine is a live rubella virus derived from an infected fetus in 1965. The virus is cultured in human fetal cells and does not pass through any nonhuman cells. It does contain an antibiotic (usually neomycin) as well as sugars and salts. The vaccine stimulates antibody production much like a natural infection, but to a lesser degree. Both natural infection and vaccine-induced immunity wane with time, and reinfection may occur. During reinfection, CRS is much less likely in vaccinated than in unvaccinated individuals. Because of the waning immunity and the possibility of reinfection, it is now recommended that children have a booster before childbearing age. This is usually provided as a second dose of MMR. Another approach is to test women of childbearing age for immunity. If they are susceptible (nonimmune), they may take a rubella booster provided that pregnancy can reliably be avoided for three months.

If a pregnant woman is inadvertently given the rubella vaccine, panic need not ensue, nor abortion. It has happened many times; there has never been a case of CRS. The rubella vaccine does not harm the fetus.

In countries that have a very high immunization rate, the vaccine is effective. After the 1965 epidemic, there was a small spontaneous drop in rubella cases, but the profound and sustained drop following the introduction of the vaccine leaves little room for doubt. There are virtually no CRS cases in the U.S. today.

Use of the rubella vaccine, however, is not appropriate in all circumstances. When there is a high rate of childhood rubella infection, CRS is infrequent because the mothers are immune by natural infection. Under those circumstances, a vaccination program less than 80 percent effective may actually increase the CRS cases because the natural cycle of contagion is interrupted and unvaccinated girls may reach childbearing age still susceptible.

Since most rubella vaccine is administered as part of MMR, it is difficult to tease out the rubella effects. But based on the best available evidence, the most common side effect of rubella vaccine is arthritis. Temporary pain, swelling, and inflammation of the joints, especially the fingers and knees, occur in up to 24 percent of adults. There have been rare cases of chronic arthritis following inoculation. Whether this is coincidence or cause and effect has been debated with some heat, especially because there have been some litigation and compensation issues. Children have minimal reactions, which may include a mild fever or rash. The most dangerous reaction is allergy to one of the vaccine components, as in the case of any other vaccine or medication.

Rarely, a low platelet blood count may occur after inoculation, but it is less frequent after getting the rubella vaccine than after natural infection.

CHAPTER 13

Polio Vaccine

CLINICAL PICTURE

Poliomyelitis, literally inflammation of the gray marrow (of the spinal cord), is commonly called polio. It had other names in the nineteenth and early twentieth centuries, including dental paralysis, infantile paralysis, teething paralysis, essential paralysis of children, regressive paralysis, and, most poetically, paralysis of the morning—after the way in which a child goes to bed apparently healthy, wakes feverish in the night, and then is unable to get up in the morning. The number of names—and there were others—reflects the confusion over the nature of the disease.

The first recorded case of polio is that of five-year-old Rumba, a Syrian boy whose history was carved in stone three thousand years ago. When he became ill, he complained of headache and pain in his right leg. Having made no improvement for some five days, his father took him to the temple, where he received the most up-to-date treatment with herbs, amulets, and secret potions. He survived. The stone tablet shows that as an adult, his right leg is shriveled and he walks with the aid of a crutch, but nonetheless he is the priestly gatekeeper for the warrior goddess Astarte, who saved his life. He is seen with his wife and young son bearing gifts of wine and fruit, and a gazelle.[1]

Although polio is known as a paralytic disease, it is actually primarily an intestinal infection that causes paralysis rarely (in less than 1 percent of cases). In fact, infection with the polio virus usually causes no symptoms (72 percent of all cases) or a minor illness (24 percent) that clears up by itself in a few days. Infected individuals may have headache, drowsiness, nausea, vomiting, or sore throat. This part of the illness has been referred to as the first hump of the disease.[2] In about 1 percent of cases, after a few days of apparent good health, a second hump appears. The fever returns but this time there is pain in the limbs and paralysis, especially of the legs. Within a few days the damage is done. If the infection reaches the base of the brain (bulbar polio), which contains the neural network controlling breathing, the patient dies unless artificial respiration is available. Some recover, but others are doomed to a miserable, short, ventilator-dependent life.[3] Other patients are left with various degrees of disability. Many, like FDR, are wheelchair-bound for the rest of their lives, subject to the associated medical and psychological complications.

We do not know how the 1 percent who become paralyzed differ from those who do not. There are some known predisposing factors, however. If the patient is harboring an incubating, unsuspected polio infection, an injection, any injection, may transform what would have been a minor illness into paralytic polio. This phenomenon, known as provocation polio, has resulted in the paradoxical situation whereby a vaccine to prevent one disease (for example, tetanus) causes another disease (paralytic polio). It is theorized that the slight injury caused by the injecting needle is sufficient to provide the virus with access to the nearby nerves and then the spinal cord. In countries that have very few cases of polio, the likelihood of provocation polio is rare, but where, as in the Third World, polio is prevalent, provocation polio is much more common. Provocation polio, unfortunately, is not restricted to natural, wild polio, but may also be associated with the oral polio vaccine, as we shall see.

Tonsillectomy is another predisposing factor. Convincing epidemiological and statistical studies show that persons who have had tonsils surgically removed, even years before, are prone to develop the most severe, bulbar form of poliomyelitis. In this case, the phenomenon is due to removal of the tonsils' powerful immune defenses.

Having survived and made substantial recovery, some patients are afflicted by the postpolio syndrome. This is a strange condition in which the symptoms and paralysis of the original illness return twenty to thirty years later. The cause of this complication has been the subject of much conjecture and theorizing, but it remains a mystery.

EPIDEMIOLOGY

Although polio is, as we have seen, an ancient disease, epidemics have occurred only since the beginning of the twentieth century. In the preindustrial era, almost the entire community became infected with the polio virus in infancy. There were relatively few paralytic cases because the newborn was partially protected by the mother's antipolio antibodies. The antibodies did not prevent infection, but did protect against the paralytic form. The virus was everywhere, but invisible.

The polio virus is spread primarily by feces: diaper-dirty hands to mouth or spoon—the so-called fecal-oral route. As public health standards improved, there was increasing concern with personal hygiene, and parents tried to keep infants and toddlers away from "dirt." This contributed to a decrease in the spread of the polio virus, so that many individuals escaped infection. These individuals remained susceptible, and when they became numerous enough, the smoldering infection ignited into an epidemic. Because the disease seemed to hit hardest at the group that was most hygiene-conscious, polio was referred to as the "disease of the middle class." An epidemic ended only when virtually the whole population became infected. In time, the cycle would repeat itself.

The epidemics began in various parts of the world at the end of the nineteenth century. The first epidemic, in the U.S. was the 1894 Vermont epidemic, in which there were 132 patients, of whom thirty were permanently crippled and eighteen died.

The 1916 New York epidemic consisted of 27,000 cases and 6,000 deaths. In his book *A Summer Plague*,[4] Tony Gould describes that frightening summer. In Europe, the Great War was grinding on. The Somme offensive started on July 1. In New York there was polio panic.

Since the polio outbreak started in the Italian community, immigrants became the scapegoats. According to the *New York Times* that same day, "There was a report . . . that the disease had been brought to America by Italian immigrants, though . . . no cases had been noticed among immigrants. . . . Quarantine had no record of epidemics in any of the towns of Italy." The commissioner of health blamed the Brooklyn citizens themselves for whatever garbage there was in their streets. "Brooklyn," he said, "had not developed sufficient pride to keep its own streets clean." Strict sanitary regulations were in force, and reports of "violations of the Sanitary Code," leading to court cases and fines, appeared in the press with regularity.

The commissioner of health admitted that "in epidemics of typhoid fever and most other diseases the health authorities know exactly what to do. But fighting infantile paralysis consists largely in doing everything in the hope that some of the measures taken will be effective."

Another indication of the panic precipitated by this latter-day plague was the wholesale exodus from the city of the children of the well-to-do. On July 5 the *New York Times* "conservatively" estimated that fifty thousand of them had been sent out of New York "to places considered safe by their parents"; and on July 7, "Reports of persons fleeing from town continue to come in." Equally panicky was the response of several neighboring states and communities, which took defensive action against the unwanted intruders. "Hoboken [New Jersey] led the way by isolating itself from the world, so far as new residents were concerned," the *New York Times* reported on July 14.

> Policemen were stationed at every entrance to the city—tube, train, ferry, road, and cow path—with instructions to turn back every van, car, cart, and person laden with furniture and to instruct all comers that they would not be permitted under any circumstances to take up their residence in the city.
>
> Cats and dogs were suspected of being carriers of the disease; strays were rounded up, and pets put down. In early July animals were being destroyed at a rate of 300 to 450 a day.

As the summer faded, so did the epidemic.

After the 1916 panic, cases remained at relatively low levels[5] until the forties and early fifties, during which decade the U.S. was ravaged by yearly outbreaks involving on the average 40,000 cases per year. The 1952 epidemic was larger even than 1916, causing 60,000 cases, but fewer deaths. After 1955, when the first widely used vaccine appeared, the number of cases dropped precipitously. There have been no major U.S. epidemics since. The last U.S. case of naturally acquired polio occurred in 1979.

THE VACCINES: SALK KILLED VIRUS (IPV)

It was the best of vaccines, it was the worst of vaccines. The vaccine eradicated polio in the U.S., but everything that could go wrong in a vaccine did go wrong. The polio vaccine story emerges from a tangle of ignorance, great science, medical practice, politics, luck, and intensely personal rivalries and jealousy. And, of course, money and power.

The bare story can be quickly told. In 1955, Jonas Salk's killed virus vaccine was licensed. It was highly effective; the number of polio cases decreased phenomenally. But multiple injections were required; these were expensive and inconvenient and resisted by portions of the population. Furthermore, some individuals did not respond to the vaccine.

Just four years later, in 1959, Sabin's live, oral polio vaccine was also approved. It largely replaced the Salk vaccine because it induced lifelong immunity, was easily administered by mouth on a sugar cube, and had the advantage of spreading to unimmunized contacts so that they too were "vaccinated."

But it was later discovered that the oral vaccine actually caused polio in a very small number of cases. That resulted in a tilt back to Salk's vaccine amid much and angry dispute about the relative merits of the two vaccines.

From 1966 to 1969 the official recommendation was to give both vaccines—first the Salk vaccine, then boosters with the oral vaccine. Ultimately the oral vaccine was abandoned; the killed vaccine is the only one available in the U.S.

Let us go back to the beginning and look at this in more detail. The story starts with Dr. Invar Wickman, who carefully observed a polio epidemic at the Stockholm Pediatric Clinic in 1905. He confirmed the long-held suspicion that polio is contagious. Even more important, he recognized for the first time that in many instances polio was a mild intestinal infection that did not cause paralysis but could be nonetheless transmitted to others. Sadly, he committed suicide at age forty-one, in 1914, but his historic monograph of 1907 earned him, along with FDR and other luminaries, a permanent place in the Polio Hall of Fame at Warm Springs, Georgia, in 1958.

Just one year after Wickman published his paper, Karl Landsteiner, an Austrian scientist, made another leap forward. He ground up a portion of the spinal cord of a ten-year-old boy who had died of polio and injected the material into the brains of two Old World monkeys. Both monkeys developed paralytic polio. Landsteiner and his colleagues also found that whatever was being transferred was much smaller than bacteria and in fact was invisible in the microscopes of the day.[6] Ultimately they demonstrated that polio is caused by a virus. They also demonstrated that the serum of monkeys that survived polio contained "germicidal substances," which we know as antibodies today. Since the researchers could grow the polio virus only in monkey neural (brain and spinal cord) tissue, many monkeys were required. These were in short supply[7] in Vienna, so Landsteiner moved his research to the Pasteur Institute in Paris, where monkeys were still available. His work was the foundation on which a vaccine would finally be built.

In 1936 there was an ultimately lethal competition between two would-be vaccine inventors, Maurice Brodie at NYU and John Kollmer at Temple University. Brodie concocted a "vaccine" from an emulsion of ground-up spinal cords of infected monkeys. He attempted to deactivate the virus by exposing the vaccine to formaldehyde, phenol, and polio antiserum. He tried the vaccine on twenty monkeys, and with that woefully inadequate experimental base conducted a human trial with three thousand children. The vaccine was of little or no value and was associated with severe side effects. His research career was destroyed, and he later killed himself.

Even worse was Kollmer's vaccine. He attempted to attenuate polio virus obtained from monkey spinal cords. He created a stew of spinal cord tissue and various chemicals and refrigerated the mixture for two weeks. He used it on a few monkeys, himself, his children, and twenty-two others. He was so convinced of the value of his vaccine that he distributed thousands of doses to physicians around the country. This vaccine caused many cases of polio, some fatal. It probably had no value as a vaccine. At a medical society meeting in 1935 he said, "I wish the floor would open up and swallow me."

What both these disasters did accomplish was to delay the development of a safe and effective vaccine. But the door was reopened by John Enders, a fighter pilot, realtor, language scholar, and ultimately virologist. In 1941, working on the mumps virus, he demonstrated two things: A killed virus could immunize an animal, and it was possible to attenuate the virus so that it was not virulent but could still elicit an immune response. The application of these two principles to the polio virus is the basis of the polio vaccines. Enders also accomplished what no one else had: He learned how to grow the polio virus in the lab. At first he used the cells of a miscarried human fetus or the cells of a prepuce obtained at circumcision. Later, monkey kidney and other tissue were used. He made it possible to grow large quantities of virus in the lab, thus solving the monkey problem

For these accomplishments, he along with his youthful associates Frederick Robins and Thomas Weller received a Nobel Prize. Enders's Nobel lecture is a study in modesty and clarity; he respected and acknowledged the work of his peers, including Salk and Sabin, both of whom stood on Enders's shoulders. Now all the pieces were in place. The frantic race to produce a vaccine was on again.

Salk won. He won the race, thanks in part to Basil O'Connor. Salk met O'Connor while returning from the 1950 Second International Poliomyelitis Conference in Copenhagen. Salk and O'Connor, the multimillionaire law partner of FDR and director of the March of Dimes,[8] became close friends. O'Connor provided Salk with massive financial aid and, when necessary, political support.

Back in the lab, Salk and his associates, using meticulously controlled conditions, were able to demonstrate that there are three different polio strains, and all could be completely killed by formalin while preserving efficacy in a vaccine. They discovered the properties of the three polio viruses and developed methods to grow the virus fast and in large quantities. To make the vaccine, virus was grown in monkey kidney cells, harvested, killed, and purified. The resulting vaccine was tested for residual live virus.

After successful experiments with monkeys in 1952, Salk injected the first human volunteers, including himself, his wife, and their three sons. By 1953, Salk had quietly done human trials in over a hundred children at the Watson School for Crippled Children and the Polk State School, a Pennsylvania facility for mentally retarded individuals. The children did develop antibodies, indicating at least some degree of immunity, and there were no adverse effects. He published this work the following year.

Salk was ready for large clinical trials, but the idea was opposed by much of the scientific community, including Albert Sabin, who was working on a live vaccine. He testified that the Salk vaccine, known also IPV (inactivated polio virus), was dangerous and should not be used. He believed that only a live virus vaccine would be protective and doubted the clinical significance of the antibodies that appeared after the IPV.

The feud between the two grew bitter. Sabin, who was generally recognized as the superior scientist, called Salk a "kitchen chemist who never had an original idea in his life." But Salk had on his side the March of Dimes, the press, and intense public pressure to field a vaccine as soon as possible. The decision was made to proceed with IPV.

The director of the trial was Dr. Thomas Francis Jr. of the University if Michigan School of Public Health. The trial, the largest of its kind ever to be conducted, included 1,829,916 children. The results were unequivocal. The vaccine was safe and effective. Efficacy was better than 70 percent, enough to prevent epidemics.

On April 12, 1955, the success was announced at a press conference. The celebrations that followed rivaled those at the end of World War II. Salk, the son of Orthodox Jewish Russian immigrants, was a hero, if not actually a savior. The many scientists in the field were not happy to learn of the trial results from the newspaper instead of professional medical journals. Salk's failure to acknowledge the work of so many others further increased a growing resentment. Enders noted that scientists always build on the work of others even though "the one who places the last stone and steps across the terra firma of accomplished discovery gets all the credit."

Within days the vaccine was licensed, and a massive immunization campaign was mounted by the March of Dimes. In 1952, the year of the initial trials in Pennsylvania, there were 58,000 cases of polio; in 1957, two years after vaccine licensure, there were 5,600 cases,

The early successes were tragically marred by the so-called Cutter Incident (see chapter 3). One of several manufacturers, Cutter produced a vaccine that contained residual live polio virus. At least 260 cases of polio were caused by the vaccine. A faulty manufacturing technique was identified and corrected, and the campaign, which had been suspended, resumed.

The Salk IPV had other problems. Immunity wore off quickly so that multiple booster shots were needed to avoid the development of an adult nonimmune group. The cost of the vaccine and boosters was high, and administering the shots added to expense and decreased acceptance. Furthermore, some individuals did not respond to the vaccine.

VACCINES: A LIVE ORAL VACCINE (OPV)

Meanwhile, the search for a live oral vaccine continued in several laboratories across the country. Albert Sabin, in 1958, was the first to develop what appeared to be a suitable vaccine. He had selected a low-virulence virus that he attenuated further by multiple passages through monkey kidney cells. Clinical trials could not be done in the U.S. because so much of the population was already immunized with the Salk IVP.

In spite of the Cold War, Sabin and Soviet Union health officials managed to work together to develop large-scale safety and efficacy trials in millions of Soviet children. It was not widely known that the attenuated viral strains developed in Sabin's laboratories at the University of Cincinnati were transformed into an oral vaccine with the help of Soviet virologists. The success of this "vaccine diplomacy" did not prevent opponents of the plan from accusing the U.S. of using the Soviets as guinea pigs on the one hand, and giving the Soviets an advantage—creating a "vaccine gap"—on the other.

The trials were a success. The vaccine (Sabin OPV) was prepared from an attenuated polio virus that was easy to grow and sufficiently attenuated to be harmless, but strong enough to establish itself in the intestine sufficiently to produce an antibody response. The recipient had only to swallow a single[9] sugar cube laced with vaccine to develop lifelong immunity. It was easy and cheap.

The Sabin OPV was licensed for general use in 1961, and within five years it was the almost excusive vaccine used in the U.S.

VAPP

Soon after the licensure and wide use of the Sabin OPV, cases of paralytic polio were found to occur after vaccine administration. Further studies confirmed that these were cases of polio caused by the vaccine. The moniker "vaccine associated paralytic polio" or VAPP was assigned.

Children who had an impaired immune system were most susceptible to this live-virus vaccine. But individuals with normal immune function were also affected. This suggested that the live vaccine was reverting to a more virulent form. Transmission of such viruses caused episodes of VAPP among household members of vaccinees. Another risk factor relates to injections of any sort (see provocation polio, above).

The risk of VAPP is generally quoted as one per 2 to 3 million doses. The risk is highest for the first dose, however, so the risk after the first dose is closer to one in 750,000. Even that number was considered small when epidemics were raging, but as the number of cases of polio fell, the significance of the VAPP cases rose. By 1980 the U.S. saw its last case of natural polio. The eight to ten cases per year since have all been due to the vaccine.

In 1996 the CDC finally changed policies and recommended the administration of two doses of IVP followed by two doses of OPV. The thinking was that the IPV would prevent VAPP. This was true, but cases of VAPP continued because nonimmune contacts who had not received IPV became infected by children who had recently received the OPV.

The recommendations were a source of much controversy. A move to discontinue OPV entirely was bitterly opposed. Politics once again influenced medical decisions when persons with VAPP began successfully suing the government for damages. The atmosphere was not exactly calmed by Salk's readiness to testify as an expert witness for the prosecution. Additional pressure came from antivaccination groups and Congress.

By the year 2000 OPV was abandoned. It is no longer available in the U.S.

SV40

In 1960, a brave researcher discovered that the monkey kidney cells being used to grow both vaccines were contaminated with a cancer-producing virus. Millions of children became infected with this virus, which causes some rare cancers in humans. See the disaster chapter. We have yet to learn the end of this story.

CONCLUSION

Polio vaccine has had a tortured history involving politics, personal ambitions, uncertain medical decisions, and finances. But it is beyond question that the eradication of polio from North America is due to the vaccines. In the tropics the issues have been different because of the all-pervasive presence of the natural virus, and because the OPV is sometimes neutralized by other viruses present in the intestine. The advantages of the OPV, including less cost, ease of administration, and contact spread make OPV the best choice in the Third World. Vigorous vaccination programs have been highly successful, and the goal of worldwide polio eradication is a dream that experts hope will come true this year.

CHAPTER 14

Flu Vaccine

Influenza, now commonly called the flu, was at one time attributed to the *influence* of the stars or planets.[1] At other times it was attributed to the *grippe* of the devil. During the great 1918 pandemic, it was called the Spanish flu.[2] Since 1933 it has been attributed to three different influenza viruses (A, B, and C).

Influenza is a disease of humans, pigs, horses, and other animals. The flu virus is also commonly found in birds, which suffer no ill effects from the infection. Humans probably acquired the infection from pigs or ducks in antiquity as measured in years, but quite recently from the perspective of human evolution. As usual, Hippocrates was the first to describe flu, the symptoms of which are known all over the world—for good reason. Millions and millions of humans have experienced the abrupt onset of debilitating fever, excruciating headache, harrowing cough, painful throat, and aching back and muscles. In uncomplicated cases, recovery follows in seven to ten days. Some patients experience a prolonged period of fatigue, lack of energy, and psychological depression. Complications include secondary bacterial infections such as ear infection, pneumonia, or sinusitis. The flu virus itself sometime causes pneumonia, which is usually fatal. Mercifully, this is a rare complication. The very young, the very old, and those with pneumonia account for the majority of the 1 percent of patients who die from the flu.

Although the mortality rate of 1 percent may seem low, the absolute number of deaths has been in the multiple millions because flu epidemics have affected a large part of the world's human population. Because flu is highly contagious and has a short incubation period, it spreads very fast, sometimes covering the entire globe in a few weeks. These worldwide epidemics are called pandemics and "are among the most vast and awe-some of all earthly phenomena."[3]

There may have been flu epidemics as early as the sixth century, but the first well-documented epidemics began in the seventeenth century. The flu has been with us ever since, never absent for more than a few decades. Epidemics of varying intensity occur almost yearly, and ferocious pandemics have erupted several times in each century. "The pandemic of 1781–2 was ... one of the greatest manifestations of disease of all history."[4] Two-thirds of Rome's population and three-quarters of Britain's became ill.

Strangely, there were only a few minor outbreaks from 1830 to 1890. But on its return in 1890, flu came with a vengeance, rolling from continent to continent, leaving 250,000 dead in Europe alone, and close to a million worldwide. By the beginning of the twentieth century, however, flu was once again considered a mild disease. The pandemic of 1918 quickly changed that view. The first wave of the pandemic arose in the United States in the spring of 1918. Ominously, many of the dead were young adults, but even so, they were few in number. However, in August a second wave came, this time with a much higher mortality rate. In some populations the infection rate was horrendous. In the Alaskan village of Teller Mission, 85 percent of the residents were dead in one week. World-wide, hundreds of millions were infected even as a third wave arose at the end of the year, finally leaving a total of 20 million dead, of which 550,000 were in the US.[5] The cause of the increasing virulence of this strain of the flu virus remains a mystery.

The last pandemic was in 1969. Since then there have been more or less yearly epidemics in the United States, causing on the average 48 million cases and 220,000 deaths each year.

THE VIRUS

Too small to be seen under even under the most powerful light microscope, the flu virus can be seen in the electron microscope. The virus is spherical and has two distinct surface configurations, called H and N antigens. The H antigen is a sharp spike that attaches to the victim's cells lining the respiratory tract. The virus then drills a hole through which it injects itself into the cell. The virus DNA makes the human cells into slaves, forced to help make innumerable copies of itself. Because of its genetic makeup, the flu virus makes many mistakes in this reproductive process. These mistakes, or *mutations*, often affect the H and N antigens so that they are constantly changing. It is this continual change that allows the virus to escape our immune defenses. In a sense, the virus's reproductive incompetence is key to its success. It is so sloppy that parts of one virus can combine with parts of another, further challenging the immune system.

The relatively minor, ongoing H and N mutations are referred to as antigenic *drift*. These mutations are responsible for the yearly epidemics, which are limited in part to lingering, partial immunity acquired in previous epidemics. This is the usual pattern for the type B virus.

Periodically a different, radical change in the virus occurs. This is usually due to the combination of a prevalent human flu virus with an animal strain, giving rise to an entirely new creature. This "new" creature may be the return of one so old that there is no immunity to it left in the population, so it looks new to the immune system.[6] It is this kind of change, referred to as antigenic *shift*, that has ignited the pandemics in the past and will do so in the future. Antigenic shift occurs only in the type A flu virus.

Pigs may be especially important in this process because they are unique in being good hosts to both human and bird influenza viruses and so may cook up a toxic genetic stew that produces new combination viruses. It has been suggested that rural intimate human-pig contact accounts for the frequent appearance of new strains in the Far East.

FLU VACCINES

To produce a vaccine, a sample of the flu virus is grown in chick cells in large sterile tanks. The virus is harvested, killed with formalin, sterilized, and preserved with thimerosal (mercury) and packaged. The final product will contain traces of chicken protein and antibiotics (usually neomycin).

Producing effective flu vaccines presents unique challenges. The early flu vaccines contained intact killed virus; these frequently caused side effects. Researchers later found that splitting the virus by dissolving its fatty outer layer with detergents and then purifying the mixture with filters decreased toxicity. The whole-virus vaccine is still manufactured, but is never given to children because of the frequent side effects. In time split-virus vaccines will probably replace the whole-virus vaccine altogether.

The viruses obtained directly from patients sometimes grow too slowly, so they are combined with a benign but vigorous rapid grower. The result is a genetically engineered, rapidly growing flu virus, which makes it possible to quickly produce the large quantities of vaccine needed to prevent or control an epidemic.

The major flu vaccine problem is, of course, to keep up with the constantly changing virus. The WHO has over a hundred laboratories all over the world constantly monitoring the prevalent flu types. About six months before the winter flu season, experts review the information and decide on the makeup of that year's vaccine, which is rushed into production. There is luck and guesswork involved; if these are favorable, a safe and effective vaccine is the result. All too often, however, a new strain appears at the last moment or an apparently docile virus turns aggressive, and the virus wins another round.

EFFICACY

How well does the flu vaccine prevent the flu? The many studies done since the 1940s have come up with results that vary from almost no effect to over 85 percent protection. This variation is due to many factors, including how good the match is between virus and vaccine; how accurately flu is diagnosed[7]; and the age and general health of the patient. Results obtained in nursing home residents will differ from those of persons living independently. Even if a vaccine does not prevent flu, it may reduce the severity; this might be demonstrated by a decrease in the hospitalization rate. An overview of clinical trials suggests that overall effectiveness is probably in the 50 percent range.

Another way to look at effectiveness is to measure antibody responses to the vaccine. Once again, there is a large range of results. Children have a less brisk response than adults, who have been primed by previous exposure to the flu and flu vaccine. Natural infection stimulates the production of specialized antibodies located in the lining of the nose and throat. These antibodies, called IgA, prevent the virus from penetrating the lining of the nose and throat. The injected flu vaccine, which bypasses this system, does not produce IgA. That is one reason researchers at the VA and elsewhere are studying nasal flu vaccines.

The duration of protection is yet another problem with the flu vaccine. Immunity after vaccination rarely lasts more than one year.

Recommendations for vaccination vary almost yearly depending on the virulence of the virus and the availability of the vaccine. In general, persons with almost any chronic disease are more susceptible to complications and death and should be vaccinated yearly. Health care workers should be vaccinated to prevent spreading infection to the patients they come in contact with. Individuals providing critical community needs should be vaccinated so that the community is not deprived of their services during an epidemic.

SIDE EFFECTS

Some of my patients refuse to take the flu vaccine because "every time I get the shot, it gives me the flu." Strictly speaking, this is not possible because the vaccine contains only killed virus, but the headache, muscle pains, joint pains, and fever that less than 1 percent of patients experience after getting the vaccine does resemble a mild case of the flu. Children are more likely to have these side effects, even with the split-virus vaccine. Pain, itching, and redness are common but harmless side effects. All these reactions are due to toxicity inherent in the viral components of the vaccine.

Patients allergic to eggs may have reactions that are on rare occasions severe. The thimerosal, formalin, and antibiotics in the vaccine may also cause allergic reactions in susceptible persons.

The swine flu fiasco of 1976 (see chapter 3) uncovered a new toxicity: Guillain-Barre syndrome (GBS), a form of paralysis that has 4 percent mortality. By January 1977 there were over 500 reported cases of GBS, with twenty-five deaths. Some 45 million doses were administered before the program was discontinued. Ironically, the feared epidemic never materialized. Since then GBS has been tracked very carefully: Since that ill-fated 1976 vaccine, the GBS rate has been one to two per million doses of vaccine.

One other adverse effect of flu vaccine is worsening of asthma.[8] This is a subject of some controversy because asthmatic children are at risk for complications of flu, so they should be vaccinated but, on the other hand, some children will have an asthma attack due to the vaccine. In the United Kingdom, immunization of children is officially recommended, but some experts do not immunize their patients.

CONCLUSION

The flu vaccine is hardly a vaccine poster child. Efficacy varies from year to year, the immunity is short-lived, mild side effects are common, and rarely, side effects may be severe. Its use in children is problematic. Epidemics have occurred, even in highly immunized populations. Nonetheless, in balance, flu immunization is, from the public health point of view, a definite plus because deaths and hospitalizations are reduced.

I expect researchers to develop better vaccines. Would that they arrive before the next pandemic.

CHAPTER 15

H. Flu (Hib) Vaccine

Hemophilus influenza infects infants and young children. It causes meningitis, brain damage, mental retardation, epilepsy, deafness, choking (epiglotitis), pneumonia, and fatal blood poisoning. The preventive vaccine is one of the best—safe and effective. Yet it is the least well known of the common immunizations. I suppose there are several reasons for this. Hib infection, while always present in the background, does not cause headline epidemics and has no famous or infamous tales associated. In addition, as vaccines go, this is a relative newcomer; the present vaccine was licensed only in 1987.

Then there is the confusion with influenza, the flu. During the 1890 flu epidemic, Dr. Richard Pfeiffer made an exciting discovery; he found a new bacterium in the throats of many flu victims. So when Pfeiffer announced his mistaken belief that his bacillus caused the flu, it was widely accepted. Pfeiffer was a luminary in Dr. Koch's Berlin lab, along with Behring, Shibasaburo, and other giants of the golden age of bacteriology.[1] He made many original and important contributions to the field, but, sadly, is best known for his biggest mistake.

It was twenty years later, during the flu pandemic of 1918, when researchers realized that Pfeiffer's bacillus was not the agent that caused flu. Influenza is caused by a virus that has no biological connection to Hemophilus influenzae.[2] The Pfeiffer bacillus's name was changed to *Hemophilus* (blood-loving), because its cultivation in the lab requires a medium that contains some components of blood, and *influenzae* in recognition of its history.

THE BUGS

Hemophilus influenzae comes in several varieties. Margaret Pitman, world-famous bacteriologist at the National Institutes of Health (NIH), discovered that there are two major forms: encapsulated and nonencapsulated. The encapsulated types are invasive and destructive. They have a bulletproof, nonstick coating: The host's white blood cells cannot get a grip on them and the chemicals of inflammation slide right off. There are six capsular types; type b is the most virulent—it is referred to as Hib. Strangely, about 3 percent of the population carry Hib in their throat without becoming ill.

There are alarming reports that this dangerous bug is learning how to resist the best antibiotics. This is a good example of "an ounce of prevention. . . ."

THE ILLNESS

The nonencapsulated forms are part of the normal flora living peacefully in the mouth of their human hosts in 75 percent of healthy children and adults. Sometimes, for unknown reasons, the bacteria become pathogens causing illnesses such as sinusitis, bronchitis, and ear infections. In adults, especially those with underlying chronic disease, the nonencapsulated strains may cause bronchitis, pneumonia, and, rarely, meningitis. There is no vaccine against these nonencapsulated bacteria, but fortunately, so far, these infections are being controlled with antibiotics.

Hib on the other hand is deadly. Before the vaccine, Hib was the most common cause of meningitis in children younger than five years, with the majority of cases occurring in the first year of life. Of the twelve thousand children per year who got meningitis, 10 percent died and 30 percent of the survivors had deafness, seizures, or brain damage. The illness starts with the child being cranky and running a fever, followed by confusion progressing to coma and death.

The list of other illnesses due to Hib include ear infections; sinus infections causing fever and congestion; epiglottitis, an inflammation and swelling of the epiglottis,[3] which can be rapidly fatal; a particularly destructive type of arthritis that occurs when blood-borne Hib lands in a joint; pneumonia and other serious lung infections; also, rarely, bone, heart, skin, and eye infections.

EPIDEMIOLOGY

Hemophilus influenzae has a strange relationship with its human host. Since man is its only host, Hemophilus influenzae can survive only because we humans allow it to. We provide room and board in the warm, moist crevices of our throats and mouth. Why do we do this? Has Hemophilus influenzae really outsmarted us and discovered the free lunch, or is there some tit-for-tat that we don't know about? Some of the bacteria that live in and on us do provide some benefits such as suppression of yeast infections, stimulation of the immune system, manufacturing of blood-clotting components, and suppression of harmful bacteria. Perhaps Hemophilus influenzae does have some hidden benefits, too. In any case, it is the healthy carrier who transmits the bacteria from person to person, allowing the infection to persist in the community. When Hib does go, for reasons unknown, on the warpath, it produces an antibiotic that kills off the unencapsulated variants so that it can invade any part of the body.

Hib infection occurs almost exclusively between the ages of two months and five years. The infant's first two months are protected by the mother's antibodies that have entered the baby's bloodstream. This protection is further increased in breast-fed babies.

Adults infrequently get Hib infection. Almost all individuals more than five years old have Hib antibodies even if they have never had Hib infection. Researchers think that some of the normal flora, such as E. coli, and some food residues resemble Hemophilus influenzae so closely that antibodies against one may be effective against the other.

THE VACCINE

Hib showed a mysterious spontaneous decline in the late 1980s. Between 1987 and 1991 the number of cases in children under five years old fell from forty to eight per 100,000. But there were still 12,000 cases of meningitis per year before the first vaccine was licensed, in 1985. Since then there has been a further 95 percent decline.

The first vaccines contained purified components of the Hib capsule and were not only ineffective, but may have even increased susceptibility.

It is difficult to immunize infants against bacteria, which have a capsule, such as Hib and pneumococcus. Most vaccines are directed at a protein on the surface of the pathogen, but these encapsulated bacteria have carbohydrate fragments on their surface. Carbohydrates stimulate the immune system less than proteins, making it more difficult to produce antibodies. The infant's immune system is not up to the job; neither cellular immunity nor antibodies are stimulated. But if the weak vaccine is conjugated ("welded") to a "carrier protein," the resulting stimulus is so strong that even the infant's immune system is alerted. The carrier protein used is a powerful stimulant, such as a fragment of tetanus toxin.

The conjugated vaccines have consistently been more effective than predicted. Since the introduction of the vaccine, cases of Hib in unvaccinated children have dropped markedly. This effect may be due to the ability of the vaccine to eliminate Hib from the healthy carrier, which is crucial for spread of the infection in the community. Hib infection has been virtually eliminated in the USA. On average, there are 300 cases per year, mostly unvaccinated children.

Three Hib vaccines are licensed for use in infants. Although there are differences in the way they are prepared, all appear to be highly effective. Head-to-head comparisons have not been done (and probably won't be done).

Some unanswered questions are: Which vaccine is best? At what age will the vaccine be most effective? How many doses is ideal, and do adults need vaccination? There is also the question of long-term safety, which only time can tell.

There are some interactions between the usual vaccines and Hib; these don't seem to be significant but are not always beneficial. There is some evidence that using different vaccines for the first and booster shots may be more effective than using the same vaccine throughout. What's special in children aged six months to two years that makes them so uniquely susceptible?

TOXICITY

The vaccines in use today have an excellent safety reputation. Since they are purified components of the bacterial cell wall, these vaccines are free of the problems associated with live or killed whole virus/bacteria.

About 5 percent of individuals have a local reaction of pain and swelling at the injection site. No serious toxicity has been established. There have been isolated reports of serious problems after vaccination, including neurological, blood platelet, and severe allergy problems. These reports are so rare that it is impossible to come to any statistically valid proof that they are or are not related to the vaccine.

CONCLUSION

The currently recommended Hib vaccines are highly effective in preventing Hib meningitis and other life-threatening infections. The safety profile is excellent.

CHAPTER 16

Pneumococcus Vaccine

The pneumococcus, known today as Streptococcus pneumonia, has probably been an intimate of our species for a very long time, but was first identified in the late nineteenth century. It was isolated from the sputum and lung tissue of patients who had pneumonia. Known as the "killer disease," pneumococcal pneumonia starts suddenly with chills, fever, headache, cough, bloody or "rusty" sputum, and chest pain. Persons who had previously been healthy usually mount an effective immune response that leads to clinical recovery during the first week or two. Persons with weak immune systems[1] are often overwhelmed by the infection and die. The pneumococcus is known as the "old man's friend" because it often ends the suffering of persons who have a terminal illness.

During that era, the turn of the nineteenth century, clinicians discovered the full spectrum of the interaction between humans and the pneumococcus. It is found in the cerebrospinal fluid of patients who have the often-fatal pneumococcus meningitis. Some survivors are left with neurological damage or convulsions. Ear infections are extremely common among infants; an appreciable number of which are caused by the pneumococcus. This can cause impaired hearing. Pneumococcus is found in arthritic joints, which usually are destroyed by the infection. In the abdominal cavity, pneumococcus causes peritonitis. Infection of the heart valves, always fatal before penicillin, is still a lethal disease. The pneumococcus is sometimes found in the bloodstream, without any source apparent. This is another often fatal complication.

Most surprising was the discovery that many perfectly healthy individuals harbor the pneumococcus in throat and nasal passages, but only a minority of these people become ill. This suggests that the pneumococcus and humans have reached an accommodation that breaks down only when bodily defenses are impaired.

The CDC estimates[2] that in the prevaccine era each year in the United States, pneumococcus disease accounted for an estimated 3,000 cases of meningitis, 50,000 cases of bacteremia, 500,000 cases of pneumonia, and 7 million cases of ear infection.

THE PNEUMOCOCCUS

While the clinicians were defining the spectrum of disease caused by pneumococcus, bacteriologists were learning its biology. It has a smooth outer capsule,[3] which eludes the grasp of the protective white blood cells and, Teflon-like, sheds attacking antibodies. Based on variations of the capsule surface, there are over ninety types of pneumococcus. To the immune system, pneumococcus looks like ninety different bacteria. The types are not all equally pathogenic, however; about ten types account for more than 70 percent of infections.

EARLY VACCINES

Researchers discovered that serum from survivors of pneumococcus pneumonia could prevent infection in rabbits and possibly in humans as well, but the results were hit or miss depending on whether or not the antiserum was the correct type. Antiserum treatment was improved by custom-making serum for each patient. This was a costly project that took days to complete and was associated with the problems that come with horse serum, from which the vaccine was derived.

The modern approach began in 1911 in South Africa. Novice workers in the gold mines there had an unusually high rate of pneumococcus pneumonia. Mortality rates were high. Researchers formulated a rather crude whole-cell vaccine. This experimental vaccine was administered to 50,000 mine workers in three years. There seemed to be some benefit, but overall the results were not very encouraging. In the 1930s a refined whole-cell vaccine containing several different types was administered to all new mine workers. Although this clinical trial would not meet today's scientific standards, there was strong evidence that the vaccine was protective. This study, in fact, is still quoted as evidence of vaccine efficacy, although it is a long way from the African gold mines of the thirties to today's USA suburbs.

In the 1940s, E. R. Squibb and Sons developed and marketed two poly-valent (containing more than one type) vaccines, one for children and one for adults. These vaccines never "caught on" and were discontinued in the fifties.

Although research into pneumococcus vaccine continued, some of the urgency was lost when sulfa and antibiotics appeared in the forties. Pneumococcus was easily killed with doses of penicillin that would be considered laughably small today. But predictably, widespread uses of penicillin allowed penicillin-resistant strains to appear. At first the resis-tance could be overcome by increasing the penicillin dose, but by the 1970s, highly resistant varieties were being found. This development redirected efforts to create a preventive vaccine.

Between 1938 and 1983, several vaccines were marketed but with-drawn because of lack of efficacy or presence of side effects. In 1983, a twenty-three-component polyvalent vaccine was licensed. Merck and Company (Pneumovax 23) and Lederle Laboratories (Pun-Immune 23) included twenty-three purified capsule components. One dose (0.5 ml) of the 23-valent vaccine contains 25 mcg. of each capsular polysaccharide antigen dissolved in isotonic saline solution with phenol (0.25 percent) or chimerical (0.01 percent) added as preservative. Many clinical trials have yielded disparate results. In spite of some encouraging field tests, this vaccine has been a disappointment. It is least effective in the very young and very old, the two groups most in need of protection. There is some dispute about the studies, but it appears that in adults this vaccine does not prevent pneumonia but does provide modest protection again the invasive, bacteremic form. This vaccine is still being used in adults and older children who are at increased risk for pneumococcus infection.

CONJUGATED VACCINES

The whole picture changed with the licensing of a conjugated vaccine (Prevnar) in the year 2000. Conjugated vaccines are similar to conven-tional vaccines, except that a carrier protein is attached to the vaccine. The carrier is a very strong immunologic stimulant,[4] which can evoke immune responses even in newborns. The current vaccine contains seven different polysaccharide antigens from different sources, which account for the majority of pneumococcus infections. Concern about the amount of car-rier is one of the limiting factors in the number of types that the vac-cine may contain. The vaccine is licensed only for children less than two years old.

EFFICACY

The vaccine is practically 100 percent effective in preventing invasive disease—primarily pneumococcus meningitis and bacteria. Efficacy in preventing ear infections is much less. This may be due in part to infection by types not covered by the 7-valent vaccine. Also, unlike vaccines, natural infection induces immune responses in the mouth and nasal passages, which limits penetration into the bloodstream.

At least one clinical study found that pneumococcus ear infections in immunized children were more likely to have one of the types not represented in the current vaccine. This situation is analogous to the development of resistance to antibiotics.

Some studies have shown that the pneumococcus vaccines may decrease the number of carriers of pneumonia. If this turns out to be the case, it will decrease the number of infections even in the immunized (herd immunity), since the symptomatic carrier is the source of most pneumococcal infections.

SIDE EFFECTS

Except for the ever-present possibility of allergy, there have been few side effects. Inflammation at the site of infection, sometimes with fever, occurs in up to 30 percent of patients; rarely, febrile convulsions occur. And, of course, there are always concerns about unknown long-term side effects; only time will tell.

CONCLUSION

A hundred years after the discovery of pneumococcus, we still are a long way from a good pneumococcus vaccine. The 23-valent type is for adults only and provides some protection against the worst forms of the disease, but does not prevent pneumonia. The conjugate vaccines for children under two have been disappointing with regard to preventing ear infection, but are effective in preventing the uncommon complications such as meningitis and bacteremia.

CHAPTER 17

Hepatitis B Virus (HBV) Vaccine

Hepatitis means inflammation of the liver. There are many causes including infection, drugs, toxins, metabolic abnormalities (congenital or acquired), and autoimmune and parasitic diseases. In this chapter we will be considering only one of the several types (A through H at last count) of viral hepatitis, hepatitis B, often referred to as HBV (hepatitis B virus).

Liver disease and jaundice have been known since antiquity, but the cause had not been identified. Hepatitis B was discovered in an unfortunate way. In 1832, Dr. Lurman of Bremen, Germany, was director of a project to inoculate 1,289 dockworkers with smallpox vaccine. Thanks to his meticulous record-keeping and sharp clinical observation, he discovered that 191 of those vaccinated (15 percent) developed jaundice weeks to months later. None of the men who had not been vaccinated became ill. It became apparent that the smallpox vaccine, which was derived from human blood plasma, had become contaminated with an agent capable of transmitting hepatitis by injection. The next major step would not come for over one hundred years.

THE ILLNESS

Hepatitis B causes a broad spectrum of illness. Some, especially children under five, may have an illness so mild that there are no symptoms, and unless blood tests are done the disease goes undetected. At the other extreme, patients may succumb in a few weeks. Still others develop chronic hepatitis that continues for decades.

The early symptoms of acute hepatitis B may include feeling "lousy," loss of appetite, and low-grade fever. Sometimes the first sign that something is not right is when someone else notices that the person's eyes are yellow. Indeed, when jaundice is severe, the yellow eyes almost glow in the dark. During this phase of the illness, the urine is usually brown and the stool pale. Almost all patients get better by themselves. A rare unlucky few who seem unable to mount a good immune defense develop fulminant hepatitis. In these cases the liver is virtually destroyed. Internal bleeding, bacterial infection, and coma are often fatal.

Following recovery from the acute phase, the illness may follow one of several paths. Some patients get entirely well and eliminate the virus, although telltale antibodies remain as a record of the infection.

Other patients become carriers of the virus. The virus lives on in the liver cells, but causes no injury to the patient, who is, however, contagious. Some carriers develop chronic hepatitis, which may be mild but often causes weakness and ill health. Sometimes the chronic hepatitis is more aggressive and progresses to cirrhosis of the liver. The liver becomes hard and shrunken due to scar tissue. These unfortunate persons eventually suffer the complications of liver failure: shriveled muscles, grossly swollen belly, and mental confusion due to an accumulation of ammonia in the brain. Death is often due to bleeding because the blood does not clot properly, and the buildup of pressure in the liver circulation causes the enlarged veins in the esophagus to rupture.

Yet another late complication of hepatitis B is cancer of the liver, an uncommon but fatal event.[1]

EPIDEMIOLOGY

Infection with hepatitis B occurs by transmission from mother to fetus or from mother to newborn; by transfusion of blood or blood products; or by contact with sexual secretions, including semen and vaginal secretions. In some cultures intravenous drug use, sexual promiscuity, and prostitution are common high-risk sources of infection. Health care workers exposed to blood, especially in dialysis centers, are also at risk.

About 90 percent of babies infected at the time of birth, or soon after, develop chronic hepatitis, presumably because they have immature immune defenses. Even though the virus remains active, these children rarely have symptoms because they do not put up a fight. Twenty-five percent of these children will, however, ultimately die of liver cancer or cirrhosis.

There are 200,000 to 300,000 new infections in the USA yearly, and there are 1 million carriers. Five thousand die of cirrhosis and 1,500 die of liver cancer.

The age distribution of hepatitis is variable. In Asia infants and children are most commonly affected, generally from the mother. In the USA infection is most common in young adults, many of whom fall into the high-risk groups.

THE VACCINE

The first immunization therapy for hepatitis B was the use of blood plasma from persons with high levels of antihepatitis B antibodies. The preparation is still used to prevent (or ameliorate) cases after known exposure to hepatitis B. Like other passive immunizations, protection lasts only as long as the donor's antibodies (usually weeks).

Experiments on human volunteers in the 1930s and 1940s proved that hepatitis was a contagious viral infection of the liver.[2] But many questions remained. Saul Krugman of New York University answered many of them during the fifties and sixties. He discovered most of what we know about hepatitis B, including route of transmission, incubation period, immune responses, and complications. His studies were done at the bucolic grounds of the Staten Island Willowbrook School for severely retarded children. At Willowbrook there was an ongoing epidemic of hepatitis, which some saw as a disgrace but which Krugman saw as a fertile field for clinical studies. He infected newly admitted children with hepatitis either by feeding them with virus from the stool of infected inmates or by injection of known hepatitis B blood products. He also treated some other newly admitted children with a prototype vaccine. He was a careful, brilliant, and thorough clinical investigator. Some of his papers are considered medical classics.

These experiments were denounced on ethical grounds, especially in the United Kingdom, but defended by Krugman, whose position was since all children at Willowbrook eventually caught hepatitis anyway, it would be for the benefit of the children in the long run, and even in the short run, because they would be housed in the well-staffed and equipped experiment suites. The counterargument was that Willowbrook could be "cured" of the hepatitis epidemic by use of standard isolation and infection-control measures. There were charges and denials regarding parents being coerced into signing consent to the experiments. At the least there were times when a child's admission was denied because the parents would not consent.

The transoceanic verbal wrestling was picked up by the media and put into political orbit. The topic was no longer hepatitis: All aspects of care were questioned. Sen. Robert Kennedy visited in 1965: He had harsh words about what he saw. Seventeen of the eighteen buildings were wrecks, conditions were deplorable, and the children were housed like animals in a zoo. Geraldo Rivera escalated the rhetoric by making comparisons to the German concentration camps. His exposé was probably the catalyst leading to a class action lawsuit that led further to an investigation of New York's care for severely impaired children. Willowbrook was finally shut down in the 1970s.

While all this was going on, future Nobel laureate Baruch Blumberg and his associates were quietly conducting some important and fascinating research that would lead directly to the hepatitis B vaccine. Blumberg was neither an infectious disease nor a liver specialist. He was interested in how a person's genetic makeup affected their susceptibility to various diseases. In the course of his medical travels, he had collected some blood from a leukemic aborigine, in which he found a previously unknown chemical that came to be called the Australia antigen (HbsAg). Curious, Blumberg found the Australia antigen in other patients who had leukemia, but also in patients who did not have leukemia. In a fascinating epidemiological "whodunit," Blumberg backtracked to the common denominator: All the patients with Australia antigen had hepatitis and had been given transfusions of blood products. In other words, Australia antigen was part of the hepatitis B virus.

Discovery of the Australia antigen immediately provided two giant steps forward: There was now a blood test to diagnose hepatitis B, and, equally important, the Australia antigen led the way directly to a vaccine. Injection of the Australia antigen induced antibodies against it, thus making the recipient immune to hepatitis B. The beauty of it was that Australia antigen, which is located on the surface of the hepatitis B virus, could be purified so that it was free of any possible contamination by other components of the virus and, of course, was not capable of causing hepatitis.

The downside of the 1980s original vaccine was that since the virus could not be grown in test tubes, it had to be prepared from the blood plasma of individuals who had recovered from hepatitis B. Such plasma could theoretically contain other unknown viruses such as HIV. Although this never occurred, it did cause some reluctance to use of the vaccine.

This problem was overcome by a feat of genetic engineering. Scientists discovered a way to genetically engineer ordinary yeast cells so that they produced Australia antigen. The vats were bubbling away, but instead of making beer, the yeast was making Australia antigen! This was cheaper and safer: no more human plasma.

EFFICACY

One measure of efficacy is to study a large population and see how well a given vaccine prevents the infection in question. In the case of hepatitis B, this kind of population study does not work because most cases are undetected until complications occur many years later.

Controlled trials have been done in highly susceptible populations with the finding of greater than 90 percent protection. There is little doubt about it—this is a highly effective vaccine. After a full series of shots, about 90 percent of persons will develop adequate antibody levels; of these there is virtually 100 percent protection from hepatitis B infection.

No one knows how long immunity induced by the present vaccination schedule will last. The antibody level drops below the critical level fairly rapidly, but even with low antibody levels, a twelve-year follow-up shows that persons immunized rarely get infected, and if they do the case is very mild. The guess is that these patients will not get the late complications.

ADVERSE REACTIONS

There have been reports of neurological complications, including multiple sclerosis. In 2002 the Institute of Medicine, after extensive review, found that there was no connection between MS and hepatitis B vaccine. This finding was based on epidemiological studies that show that MS occurs just as often in persons who have not received the vaccine. With regard to Guillain-Barre syndrome, there is not enough evidence one way or another to decide.

As always, allergies are possible and there have been dangerous anaphylactic reactions, but there are no recorded deaths.

The initial vaccines contained mercury as a preservative. Immunizing newborns with hepatitis B vaccine was loading up babies with potentially toxic levels of mercury. The CDC denied this but recommended nonetheless that mercury be removed from the vaccine. Vaccines available in the USA are now free of mercury, although mercury-containing vaccines are used extensively in other parts of the world. The mercury is needed to maintain sterility of the vaccine in multidose vials. Single-dose vials do not need the mercury but are more costly per shot than are multidose vials.

IMMUNIZATION STRATEGIES

On its first introduction into the medical community and the general public, there was considerable resistance to the use of the vaccine. The association of hepatitis B with gays, whores, and addicts did not make the vaccine especially popular, and many parents (and doctors) considered themselves and their children at low risk. The initial recommendation therefore was to vaccinate those in the high-risk categories. But except for health care workers, this group was hard to reach, and many of them had contracted hepatitis B at an early age. This approach failed to decrease hepatitis B infection and complications.

The next strategy was to immunize all adolescents. This too failed. Adolescents don't like going to the doctor and are suspicious about things like hepatitis vaccine and abstract, theoretical concerns about the future. The current strategy is to immunize all newborns before discharging them from the hospital. Once this goal is met, we can expect to see the disappearance of acute hepatitis and hepatitis B, cirrhosis, and liver cancer.

CHAPTER 18

Hepatitis A (HAV) Vaccine

INTRODUCTION

Hippocrates was, of course, the first to describe what was probably hepatitis—it was called epidemic jaundice. These were the days when illness was classified as a disturbance of the balance among the four humors: yellow bile, black bile, blood, and phlegm.

Jaundice is the clinical hallmark of inflammation of the liver. The liver normally clears the blood of bile pigments, but in hepatitis it is unable to keep up, so the pigments accumulate and are deposited in the skin and other tissues. The jaundice is best seen in the white of the eye. In heavily pigmented persons, jaundice may be best visible under the tongue. The examination should be done in daylight; beware of the yellow curtains favored by emergency rooms.

In addition to hepatitis, there are myriad causes of jaundice. For example, excessive breakdown of blood can overload the liver, as in sickle cell anemia. A gallstone or cancer can block the bile ducts, causing the pigment to be retained. Translated into med-speak, we have noted three kinds of jaundice: hepatocelluar disease (hepatitis), hemolytic (anemia), and obstructive jaundice (gallstone).

There are (by last count) seven types of viral hepatitis, A to G. A, B, and C are the most common. B and C have a propensity for cirrhosis, liver failure, and death. HAV is a lot less unfriendly. Almost everyone recovers, and there is no chronic form. There are vaccines only against HAV and HBV. HAV is a picornavirus (RNA). It is similar to the polio virus.

HAV

For centuries, HAV has been the soldiers' unwelcome but constant companion. In World War II, in the Mediterranean basin, 9 percent of troops were disabled by HAV at any given time. Great Britain and the Allies provided support to researchers to get control of the disease. McCollum and Bradley in the United Kingdom and Neefe and Havens in the United States found that HAV could not be transferred to laboratory animals. Humans were to be the experimental animal of choice. Human volunteers ingested bacteria-free filtrates of diarrhea stool and also drank from a well contaminated with HAV. At least some of the volunteers were the investigators themselves. These experiments defined the mode of transmission, incubation period, chronicity, and other clinical features of HAV. Meanwhile, Krugman was studying the natural history of the diseases, and in a series of controversial papers he described the Willowbrook experiments and the early use of gamma globulin.

HAV: THE ILLNESS

Two to six weeks after exposure to HAV, the symptoms begin. The incubation period depends on the size of the HAV dose: the larger, the shorter. The illness begins with flulike symptoms, including fever, aches and pains, and feeling sick. The appetite goes,[1] and the patient complains of nausea and may have vomiting. As the skin turns yellow and the urine brown, the stool becomes light in color. A rash and joint pains may occur after about ten days. Recovery usually takes two to three weeks, but some patients have recurrent symptoms for months and suffer from a prolonged period of fatigue. A very unlucky few develop fulminant hepatitis. The liver literally disappears, and the patient becomes demented or delirious (hepatic encephalopathy). The skin is deep yellow, almost brown, and fragile. There is bleeding from every orifice. The patient can't and doesn't want to eat. A liver transplant may be the only chance for survival. The cause of fulminant hepatitis is unknown, but it usually occurs in older patients.

EPIDEMIOLOGY

HAV is transmitted via the fecal-oral route, as when a wriggly baby is being inexpertly diapered, but the transmission is usually less obvious.

Infected food-handlers who don't wash their hands real well after using the toilet are one source of epidemics. Most often the source, as in this case, is contaminated food or water. The virus is hardy and can survive for a month in the environment.

Patients are most contagious early in the incubation period until about a month after the onset of the illness. Patients are contagious weeks before they aware of being infected.

The great green onion epidemic in Monaca, Pennsylvania, in 2003 is a good example of an HAV epidemic. In October and November 2003, 555 persons became ill with HAV. An epidemiologic investigation found that all the patients had eaten at one particular restaurant during a four-day period. Individuals developed symptoms two to six weeks later (the usual HAV incubation period). Thirteen restaurant employees had HAV but were ruled out as the epidemic source because they became ill at the same time as the patrons. Two hundred ninety-seven patrons were interviewed in detail. All had eaten menu items containing scallions. Here, so you can get the flavor of the investigation, is an excerpt from the report:

> Interviews conducted at Restaurant A, food service workers described green onion storage, washing, and preparation practices. Green onions were shipped in 8.5-lb. boxes containing multiple small bundles (6–8 green onions per bundle). Each box was unpacked, and bundles were stored upright (root side down) and refrigerated in a bucket with ice included in the shipment. Green onions were stored [five days or less] before processing, which consisted of rinsing intact onion bundles, cutting the roots off, and removing the rubber bands. Green onions from each box were chopped by machine to yield approximately 8 quarts. Chopped green onions were refrigerated for approximately 2 days.

The green onions were backtracked to Mexico. Three persons died. The restaurant is closed.

This case typifies one type of spread of HAV. In this case the food handlers were not the source of the epidemic. The occurrence of HAV disease is high in low-tech societies. Almost all children become infected, but most do not become ill. There is a direct correlation between the patient's age and the severity of the illness. Ninety-five percent of children under five years old are asymptomatic (silent). By age fifteen, 25 percent have symptoms, while the rate is 90 percent in adults. Paradoxically, as hygiene improves, the number of cases rises. We have seen this repeatedly; where hygiene is poor, children get infected at an early age but the infection is silent. As environmental conditions improve, more adults are susceptible. This is bad in two ways. If an adult becomes infected, the disease is likely to be severe. Furthermore, if the nonimmune population gets large enough, herd protection may be lost and epidemics occur.

There are over thirty thousand cases of HAV infections per year in the USA. One hundred die. At risk are household contacts, travelers, residents in nursing homes, day care centers, certain susceptible communities (including Inuit, Native American, and Pacific Islander children), jails, persons with chronic liver disease (HAV superimposed on patients with chronic liver disease have a 40 percent mortality), men who have sex with other men, commercial sex workers, and street drug users.

IMMUNIZATION

During World War II, scientists learned how to extract immune globulin (gamma globulin) from human blood serum. This work was a spinoff of the study of shock in the injured soldier. This immune globulin fraction of serum contains the donor's antibodies. If an individual had hepatitis and recovered, there would be antihepatitis antibody in the immune globulin. Researchers soon found that an injection of immune globulin would protect the recipient from HAV infection, but this lasted for a few months at best. As such it was not practical on the battlefield. But it is used even now as pre-exposure prophylaxis for the traveler who may be exposed to HAV. The HAV vaccine is better, but the immune globulin works immediately, whereas the vaccine takes two to four weeks to raise antibodies to protective levels. Immune globulin is also used for post-exposure prophylaxis for persons who have been exposed through close contact with an infected individual or eaten contaminated food. The immune globulin must be administered within two weeks of exposure. It prevents hepatitis altogether or, sometimes, allows a mild case through.

In order to make various batches equally potent, each is made from literally thousands of donors. This is immediately alarming, but there have been no instances of the immune serum carrying any pathogen into a recipient. The serum is tested for HIV and other blood-borne infections.

The first vaccine against HAV was licensed in 1995. There are now two vaccines available, Haavrix and VAQTA. Both are whole-virus formalin-killed preparations. The viruses are grown in human cells and contain adjuvants.

Postvaccination antibody levels have been very high, and extensive field tests have shown excellent protection rate. Universal vaccination has not been recommended unless the incidence goes over twenty cases per 100,000 population, about twice the number in the U.S. The vaccine is recommended for travelers visiting endemic areas (Central and South America, Africa, the Middle East, and Asia) and for IV drug users, multiple sex contacts, and members of ethnic groups that have a high incidence of HAV infection.

There are no serious side effects, but pain at the injection site, headache, and fever occur occasionally. The vaccine is not licensed for children under two years of age. Children under two do not respond well to the vaccine, possibly because of maternal antibodies.

CONCLUSION

HAV vaccines are among the newest. In the USA, disease occurrence is very low, and there are no serious or chronic complications except for the extremely rare episode of fulminant hepatitis. HAV infection has characteristics that make it a candidate for eradication. Humans are its only host, diagnosis is not difficult, and the use of immune globulin and HAV vaccines can be effective.

At this time, however, an HAV eradication program does not have a high priority in the developed countries (where there are so few cases) or in developing countries (which have other priorities, including TB and HIV).

CHAPTER 19

BCG: The Hunt for a TB Vaccine

The inability to control tuberculosis throughout the world represents the most colossal failure of public health service in human history.[1]

INTRODUCTION

In 1802 the inimitable Robert Koch discovered the organism that causes most cases of tuberculosis, Mycobacterium tuberculosis. Immediately, the hunt for a vaccine was begun. The first and only one to be used clinically was BCG, named for its developers, Calmette and Guerin. Four billion doses have been administered since 1921, but we still do not know how it works or even if it works. BCG has been used all over the world except for the USA and the Netherlands. In the mid-nineteenth century, the death rate in America was 400 per 100,000 population. By 1950 the number of deaths in the eastern U.S. had fallen to twenty-six per 100,000. In 2001 in the USA there were only 5.6 cases per 100,000—an all-time low. But now a new epidemic, possibly worse than any before, is slowly tramping across the globe. Worldwide, 2 billion persons (a third of the world's population) have latent infection.

HISTORY

Archaeological evidence suggests that TB has been with us for five thousand years. An Egyptian mummy dated to 3000 B.C. shows what is said to be clear evidence of TB of the bones. In China a mummified body from the early Han dynasty (206 B.C.–A.D. 7) shows tuberculosis scars in the lungs. Native American skeletons dating back to 800 B.C. show signs of TB. A Chilean mummy of A.D. 290 still had identifiable tuberculosis in her lungs.[2] This and other evidence suggests that TB was worldwide in pre-historic times. Epidemics arose not because bacteria were introduced to a "virgin" population, but from changes in the host population and its environment.

Hindu, Babylonian, Chinese, Greek, and Roman texts described tu-berculosis and recommended treatments. Homer, Hippocrates, and Galen discuss various manifestations of TB, often called phthisis. Even then it was noted that TB was more common in urban areas than in sparsely populated rural areas.

By the twelfth century, Taoist priests postulated the presence of ani-malcule, which attack weak individuals. TB animalcules were said to pass thorough six stages, the last of which was highly contagious.[3]

During the sixteenth and seventeenth centuries in Europe, the conta-gious nature of TB was confirmed. By the eighteenth century some autopsy series showed virtually 100 percent exposure to TB. By the nineteenth century, massive epidemics had Philadelphia, New York, London, Paris, Tokyo, and other large cities in its iron grasp. In the early nineteenth cen-tury, Europe had seventy deaths per 100,000 persons. Long before antibi-otics or vaccines appeared on the scene, the rate of TB deaths mysteriously decreased rapidly. This has been attributed to improving socioeconomic conditions in Europe and the USA. By 1950 the death rate had fallen to twenty-six per 100,000 population.

Hermann Braymer, a botany student, became infected with TB in the 1850s. His physician recommended a climate change, so Hermann moved to the Himalayas, where he collected plant specimens. He had fresh air, exercise, rest, and little stress. When he came home, he was cured. He decided to go to medical school. When he completed his studies in 1854, he established the first sanatorium. Soon the idea that fresh air, rest, good food, and contemplation could effect a cure was widely accepted. Sana-toria sprang up like mushrooms after rain. Hotel-like lodges were built on bucolic sites, where the guests who could afford it stayed for months or years.

During the one-hundred-year life of the sanatorium movement, made forever unforgettable by Thomas Mann's *The Magic Mountain*,[4] tuber-culosis was seen as a stigma, similar to cancer or mental illness today. At the same time, however, there was a romantic element to TB. Who has not wept at the deathbed of Mimi, or Violetta? TB seemed to select some of the most gifted: Chekhov, Chopin, and the Brontë sisters, Kafka, Keats, all died of TB between 1821 and 1924.

Some got better and many died. A particularly unlucky group was deemed suitable for collapse therapy. The physician would inject air into his patient's chest, causing the lung to collapse. Since the lung re-expanded rapidly, the procedure had to be done many times. In some cases the ribs were actually removed, causing the entire side of the chest to cave in. The resulting deformity was hard to hide.

In addition to the grand, spa-like sanatoria, some health departments set up little cottages where patients could rest, sleep, and stroll about. The "movement" of sanatoria had its outspoken critics, but the arguments became moot upon the arrival of streptomycin and other antibiotics. The sanatoria had had their day. Some became hospitals, nursing homes, or dwellings. Some were simply abandoned to become the "haunted hospital" of the neighborhood.

THE ILLNESS

Tuberculosis takes many forms—from the persons who never knew they were infected to the victims who died only after enduring decades of misery.

TB is transmitted by the aerosolized droplets coughed[5] up by an individual who has active tuberculosis. Even one bacterium inhaled by a person within range of the cough may be infectious. Before pasteurization of milk, Mycobacterium bovis caused many cases of intestinal tuberculosis.

In areas where TB is prevalent, children are infected at an early age. They may have no symptoms or, more commonly, have a mild illness, perhaps with a cough or fever. During this time, the bacteria are seeded throughout the body. In most cases the child's immune system soon walls off and controls the spread, but some bacteria survive for the life of the host. A chest x-ray would show swollen glands in the chest, and later a little fleck of calcium in the upper lobe will tell the tale many years later.

Sometimes the immune system is unable to contain the primary infection. All organ systems become impaired and the patient may die in a matter of weeks. If the immune system does wall off the bacteria, they may escape at some time in the patient's life when immunity is impaired. Old age, cancer, cancer therapy, HIV infection, alcoholism, and lack of needed medical attention are some causes of impaired immunity. Left untreated, the victim gets sicker and sicker, coughing up blood, running fevers, losing weight. Shortness of breath gets progressively worse and "tuberculomas," cancerlike nodules, may appear anywhere on the body.

If located in the brain, this is often the immediate cause of death. Meningitis is another fatal neurological complication.

NEW EPIDEMIC

The new antituberculosis drugs changed everything. Cure was possible. As we noted, the sanatoria were closed, putting some still ill patients in the street. The strong public health clinics, the mobile chest x-ray programs, some social services, and follow-up of contacts all began to deteriorate as public interest in TB faded. At first the number of TB cases continued to fall, but in 1980 the case level stabilized and then began to increase. Between 1985 and 1992 there was a 20 percent increase in the number of cases. This increase was attributed to outbreaks in prisons and nursing homes, the HIV epidemic, homelessness, emigration, and drug use. Since 1992, however, there has been a decline again in the USA and other industrialized nations. This has been attributed to revitalized public health measures.

In Asia, Africa, and to some extent the former Soviet Union, TB is out of control. Traditional public health measures are failing because of wars, poverty, and social disorganization. The HIV and TB epidemics reinforce each other; coinfection is becoming common and progresses rapidly.

Even more frightening is the development of multiresistant strains of TB. M. tuberculosis knows how to become resistant to single drugs, but multiple drugs will usually outwit it. Resistance occurs when treatment is erratic or prematurely discontinued, or if only one or two drugs are used when the clinical situation calls for three or more. These strains are resistant to all antibiotics. Infection by one of these organisms is usually fatal.

Social chaos, HIV, and multidrug-resistant TB are creating a deadly environment that could cause the worst epidemic in human history. We have the tools and knowledge to control TB, but delay in their use may be deadly.

CONTROL AND PREVENTION

TB is a preventable disease. Tracing the contacts of patients who have the active disease is the critical first step. The initial interview will define the intensity of exposure. Is the active case a household member, a schoolmate, a close sleepover friend, a grandparent?

The second step is the TB skin test (PPD). A positive test is an immune response indicating the presence of M. tuberculosis. A "false" negative test may occur during the incubation phase or in the patient who has immune impairment or overwhelming TB. If the skin test is negative, the patient should start INH antituberculosis therapy. If the test remains negative at three months, the medication can be discontinued. A case of TB has been prevented.

If the skin test is positive, the patient should be treated. The treatment regimen should be individualized based on degree of exposure, the skin test, chest x-ray, and other factors. The treated individual is no longer contagious within weeks of starting treatment, and a cure can be expected.

As noted, it is vital that the patient follow the assigned regimen, but some patients have difficulty taking their medication. In such cases, DOT (direct observation therapy) may improve results. DOT is defined as delivery of every dose of medication by a health care worker who observes and documents that the patient actually ingests or is injected with the medication. Delivery alone to the patient without observation and documentation is not DOT.

VACCINE

In 1908, Albert Leon Charles Calmette and Camille Guerin began a search for a TB vaccine. They were well suited for this task. Calmette was a naval physician and traveled widely, meeting many scientists in the forefront of microbiology. His early work involved snake antivenin and a variety of biological poisons. Guerin, on the other hand, was a veterinarian with much experience with M. bovis (cow tuberculosis). Guerin obtained a specimen of M. bovis from a cow that had M. bovis mastitis and cultured it in the lab. The hope was to attenuate and modify the M. bovis to the point that it was not harmful but could induce immune (antibody) responses when administered. They kept a continuous culture of this organism for 231 cycles in thirteen years, from 1908 to 1921. At that point, they believed that they had finally succeeded in developing a safe and effective vaccine against TB. It was a live vaccine derived from cow tuberculosis. The bacterium at the end of the thirteen years of manipulation needed a new name: BCG.

What followed was strange. In 1948 the first international BC Congress endorsed the vaccine, and WHO and UNICEF organized campaigns for mass childhood vaccination, though there was virtually no clinical data to prove efficacy. There were no controlled clinical trials; there weren't even any uncontrolled trials. Efficacy was based on animal data and skin test conversion. Every year 100 million children were vaccinated; more than 4 billion doses have been administered.

Many field trials were done between 1935 and 1975, but they were beset with problems. Researchers had to recruit thousands of patients if the results were going to bear the scrutiny of statisticians. For the same reasons, the study subjects would have to be followed up for years or decades. If active TB or overall death rates were the end points, such a study would obviously be very expensive.

There were all kinds of controlled and uncontrolled biases. Asians and Native Americans are congenitally more susceptible to TB infection and may respond differently. Some study sites had more nontubercular mycobacterium in their environment than others.[6] The BCG was different from site to site. Diagnostic criteria varied from study to study.

Some variation from one clinical study to another is to be expected. The range of results of these studies, however, went from less than zero protection (the BCG appeared to *increase* the number of cases) to about 70 percent protection.

Clinicians, professors, pathologists, and statisticians analyzed, reanalyzed, dissected, inspected, and rejected the studies. There was consensus on some points. Sometimes the BCG worked and at other times it did not. It did not prevent primacy infection. That is to say, a person could "catch" TB if they were within range of the patient's cough.

CONCLUSION

In the past, and probably even now, TB was and is a curable infection that could be controlled with screening skin tests and chest x-rays accompanied by aggressive follow-up. In the USA, TB is present only in the socially marginal groups[7] that are largely out of sight. Also out of sight is a TB epidemic in progress. Thirty percent of the human population is infected, most of whom do not have symptoms. The worldwide HIV epidemic is feeding the TB epidemic. HIV weakens the immune system, which activates the latent TB, which in turn infects the vulnerable HIV-positive population. The cycle can still be broken by old and simple measures, but only if there is some degree of social stability and a reasonably effective public health system. If we let the multidrug-resistant TB germs loose, the consequences are not hard to imagine.

BCG can provide some protection against the lethal meningitis, military spread, and other complications, but it cannot prevent the spread of TB infection and so is of only marginal use.

PART 3

Special Vaccines

CHAPTER 20

Anthrax Vaccine

THE ILLNESS

Anthrax is an infectious disease that would be of interest primarily to biblical scholars[1] and large-animal veterinarians but for its potential as an instrument of bioterrorism. Anthrax is caused by the bacterium Bacillus anthraces. Its natural hosts are domestic and wild herbivores, including alpaca, camels, and sheep. Angora goats most commonly carry the bacterium. Humans become infected through contact with the hide of these animals, giving rise to such names for the illness as "wool-sorter's disease," "rag picker's disease," and "malignant pustule." Other industrial exposures include handling bristles for brushes or making buttons out of animal horns or butchering contaminated meat.

Almost all of the infections are of the easily cured cutaneous form, affecting the skin. A few days after contact with a contaminated hide, a blister develops, then an open sore with a black[2] base. Without antibiotic treatment, the infection can be destructive, spreading deep into the tissues and the lymph nodes.

Much less common, but lethal when it occurs, is the pulmonary form that affects the lungs. The illness starts out like a cold or the flu but progresses rapidly to a deadly penetration into the chest. Unless treated at the earliest stage, the afflicted die.

There is also a gastrointestinal form, which is rare in humans in the USA.

BACILLUS ANTHRACES

B. anthraces was the first bacterium proven to cause a disease. The great Robert Koch performed the critical experiments and observations. Using

B. anthraces, he even developed the first live attenuated vaccine. This type of vaccine is still used in veterinary practice.

B. anthraces has a strange life cycle. When exposed to oxygen, it forms a microscopic, lumpy spherical spore that has a multilayered, tough protein shell to protect its precious DNA cargo. The spores can lie dormant for decades. When, finally, they find a break in the skin of a victim or are inhaled or swallowed, the host's defensive white blood cells attack the spores but succeed only in removing the shell and freeing the DNA to produce the virulent bacteria. The bacteria make short work of the infected animal, which decomposes rapidly, exposing the bacteria to oxygen which stimulates spore formation, completing the life cycle.[3]

Anthrax is so spectacularly lethal because it fools the immune system and because it releases three different toxins, each poisonous in its own right.

Anthrax occurs in epidemics in animals all over the world. There have been major anthrax die-offs: 60,000 cattle in Europe in the seventeenth century ("black bane disease"); a million sheep in Iran in 1945; 6,000 cases in Zimbabwe.

In times of drought, cattle crop their feed close to the grassland, increasing inhalation exposure. In times of flood the spores are brought to the surface, increasing ingestion exposure.

THE VACCINE

The vaccine licensed for humans, manufactured by the Michigan Biologic Institutes, is made from an attenuated, weakened anthrax strain that does not form spores. The vaccine is prepared by filtering the soup in which the bacteria are grown. No living organisms are in the vaccine, which does contain aluminum hydroxide, formaldehyde, and benzethonium. The content or structure of the active components of the vaccine have never been identified. The potency of each lot of vaccine is crudely measured by injecting vaccine into guinea pigs.

The recommended schedule is to give doses at zero, two, and four weeks, with booster shots every year.

Side effects include mild to severe swelling and pain at the injection site in 2 to 3 percent of vaccines. About 1 percent have mild flulike reactions. Reports of serious neurologic and other complications associated with anthrax vaccination during the first Gulf War have not been scientifically verified.

EFFICACY

Estimates of clinical efficacy depend on one controlled clinical trial involving workers in four Northeastern USA mills that processed raw goat hides contaminated by B. anthraces. The vaccine used was an experimental one and differs from the currently used strain. The current strain has never been subjected to a controlled clinical trial. In the goat-hide trial, the vaccine was found to be very effective against the cutaneous form. Since almost all of the cases were the cutaneous type, there was no useful information about efficacy against the more serious inhalation form of anthrax.

The vaccine does stimulate antibodies and is effective in monkeys and other animals, but the relevance of these data to current anthrax bioterrorism issues is questionable.

The vaccine was initially licensed for protection against the cutaneous form of anthrax. Routine use of the vaccine is recommended for individuals who have a potential exposure to it in industry, veterinary medicine, and agriculture.

PUBLIC HEALTH AND MILITARY ISSUES

Anthrax has the potential for creating a human and ecological disaster. As we have seen, anthrax in nature is usually limited. Control of anthrax in cattle and immunization of exposed workers further limits its spread. Widespread dispersion of spores, however, could be a nightmare.

Fearing possible German germ warfare during World War II, the British experimented with the use of anthrax spores as a weapon. They dropped anthrax bombs on the idyllic island of Gruinard in the Hebrides. All the sheep on the island died, and it was fifty years before it was safe for humans to even walk the land. And this in spite of attempts to remove the spores using 280 tons of formaldehyde diluted in 2,000 tons of seawater.

On April 2, 1979, there was a strange outbreak of anthrax in the former Soviet Union city of Sverdlovsk, home of a military microbiology laboratory. Of ninety-four people known to have been affected, at least sixty-four died. Officials attributed the epidemic to ingestion of contaminated meat, but the location and timing of the cases suggested otherwise. Thirteen years later, Yeltsin admitted that the epidemic was due to a faulty filter that allowed release of spores into the atmosphere.

The latest use of anthrax as a weapon was the October 2001 attempt to kill Senate majority leader Tom Daschle and Senate Judiciary Committee chairman Patrick Leahy. The mailings, contaminated with anthrax spores, killed five people, sickened many others, and virtually shut down the government for days. Anthrax has the potential for being truly a weapon of mass destruction.

In view of the threat of germ warfare during both Gulf Wars, the military required all personnel to receive the anthrax vaccine. Those who refused were punished or discharged. Six soldiers brought the issue to court on the relatively narrow argument that, since the vaccine was approved for the prevention of cutaneous anthrax, its use to prevent inhalation anthrax was an experiment, which required consent of the participant. On December 22, 2003, Judge Emmett Sullivan accepted that argument and issued an injunction halting the vaccination program that was begun in 1988.

The FDA moved, for once, with lightning speed, stating eight days later that the vaccine was safe and effective for prevention against all forms of anthrax.[4] Sullivan reluctantly lifted the injunction on January 7, and the immunization program was immediately resumed. But on October 28, 2004, however, the judge set aside a final ruling and order by the FDA that the vaccine was safe and effective. "By refusing to give the American public an opportunity to submit meaningful comments on the anthrax vaccine's classification (*safe and effective versus experimental*), the agency violated the Administrative Procedures Act." Sullivan told the Food and Drug Administration to reconsider the issue after an appropriate public comment period. "Congress has prohibited the administration of investigational drugs to service members without their consent. This court will not permit the government to circumvent this requirement," he wrote. Again, the mandatory vaccination program was suspended.

CONCLUSION

Anthrax as a "natural" disease has drawn little interest; it is not a major public health problem. Anthrax as a weapon, however, evokes fear of populations decimated, cities abandoned by the survivors of an attack. It may make sense, then, to advocate use of a preventive vaccine. Unfortunately, the only licensed human vaccine is a crude one that has never been tested in field conditions. Major questions about efficacy and long-term toxicity remain unanswered.

CHAPTER 21

Special Vaccines for Travelers, Health Care Workers, and Military Personnel

VACCINES FOR INTERNATIONAL TRAVEL

International travel is increasing rapidly for business, education, tourism, and emigration. The number of international trips is in the billions; Africa, East Asia, and the Pacific are catching up with Europe and the Americas as favored destinations.

Travel immunization should be part of the planning of every trip.[1] The first step is to make sure that you are up-to-date on the serious routine illnesses: diphtheria, measles, pertussis, and polio.

The second step will be to consider special vaccines. Making the right decisions about pretravel vaccination is an individual matter; a rote selection of vaccine depending on the destination may be inadequate. The devil is in the details. Aside from the destination, what will be your exposure? Will you be in a modern city with good water, or in a Third World country with possibly contaminated water? Will you be in the bush on an adventure tour or in the field hiking? With whom and how closely will you be interacting? Will you be doing medical, veterinary, or missionary work? Will you be in contact with animals?

Your external environment is important. So is your internal environment. Is there any indication that you have any sort of immune deficiency or chronic disease such as heart failure or liver cirrhosis? What medications are you taking, and might they interfere with your vaccination program?

If you are going to need pretravel vaccination, start weeks if not months before the departure date. Active immunization with vaccines takes weeks to be effective, and if there is more than one vaccine that has to be given in tandem, this will slow the process even more. If you don't have enough time to get vaccinated adequately, you may be able to receive immune globulin containing antibodies to the disease in question. Immune globulin provides immediate but transient protection and may interfere with other vaccines.

By the time you read this, polio may have been eradicated, although some Indian communities have refused immunization, setting back the eradication timetable.

Measles is present in Europe and Asia. You should take a course of MMR if you do not have documentation of adequate immunization. Tetanus immunity falls in time, so you should get a booster every ten years. The tetanus toxoid is administered combined with diphtheria toxoid. In recent years there have been epidemics of diphtheria in Russia, so the combination is fortunate.

Hepatitis B is prevalent in many parts of the world, so if you expect to be in Africa or northern South America for more than six months, or if you have risk factors for hepatitis and have not already been immunized, you should get the three-shot series. Since the last is given four months after the second, this has to be planned well in advance.

Hepatitis A is the most common preventable disease vaccine among travelers. The inactivated virus vaccine is clearly safe and effective. It may be underutilized in part because, unlike hepatitis B, hepatitis A is usually mild and has no chronic complications. Many persons are immune because of an hepatitis A infection that was not diagnosed. If you are going to a high-risk environment, you might want to have a blood test to see if you are immune, in which case of course vaccination is unecessary.

Typhoid fever is the second most common preventable infections vaccine among travelers. Untreated, typhoid fever can be fatal. The disease is most common in Third World societies and in parts of the former Soviet Union. Travelers to these areas should be immunized. There are two vaccines available in the USA. One is a live, attenuated bacterium. Side effects are minimal, but as in the case of any live vaccine, it should not be administered to someone who is immunosuppressed. The other vaccine is an injectable, killed virus preparation. Each is about 70 percent effective in the field. Side effects are minimal.

Meningitis is epidemic in sub-Saharan Africa. Vaccination is usually recommended if you will be staying in the area for a long time and have close contact with the local population.

Rabies (see below) immunization may be recommended for local travel in areas where rabies is common in dogs: Asia, South America, and Africa. Vaccination is especially recommended for people hiking, spelunking, camping, and doing any other activity likely to result in exposure to dogs, bats, raccoons, skunks, cats, or other carnivores.

Yellow fever is caused by a virus that is transmitted by the mosquito A. egypti, which is widely dispersed in the tropics. Yellow fever is a dangerous infection that brings with it a significant mortality rate. Unfortunately, the vaccine, an injected attenuated live virus, has in recent years caused some severe reactions, including death. Only those travelers at high, unavoidable risk of getting mosquito bites should be vaccinated. Some countries will not permit entry without a valid international certificate of vaccination if he or she has visited any country either known or thought to have yellow fever virus. Such requirements may be strictly enforced, particularly for persons traveling from Africa or South America to Asia. The vaccine is available only in yellow fever centers, which administer the vaccine and issue the certificate.

There are many (over a hundred) other vaccines not routinely recommended because the disease is rare or the vaccine is dangerous. You should plan for your trip as early as possible. Start your education at the CDC website, then consult with a physician experienced in diseases of travelers.

OCCUPATIONAL VACCINES

If you are a health care worker, you have two reasons to scrutinize your vaccination status. One reason is that you might be at risk of becoming infected; another is that you might be a hazard to your clients. Measles, mumps, German measles (rubella), and chicken pox are of particular concern. All are highly contagious and more severe in adults than in children. If your immunity has worn off, you may be at risk. On the other hand, if you are in the presymptomatic phase of any of these infections, you may infect your charges. The same logic would argue for yearly flu vaccination.

If you may possibly come in contact with blood (as a health care worker, police officer, firefighter, or laboratory technician), it is vital that you have immunity to hepatitis B. The law requires employers of health care workers to provide hepatitis B vaccination, but does not require it.

As for rabies, if you are a high-risk professional such as veterinarian, hunter, animal control officer, mail carrier, speleologist, or worker in a laboratory that contains the rabies virus, you should be vaccinated against this horrible, ancient fatal infection.

If you are in the armed forces, you may be required to receive vaccines for illnesses associated with bioterrorism or with the country where you are stationed.

CHAPTER 22

Japanese Encephalitis Vaccine

INTRODUCTION: THE PLAGUE OF THE ORIENT

Japanese encephalitis (JE) is a viral infection of the brain transmitted to man by a mosquito. There are six other types of viral encephalitis,[1] but a vaccine is available for only the Japanese variety. JE is one of seventy viruses that comprise the Genus Flavivirus. The virion is a small but complex structure. It is readily grown in tissue culture in a variety of arthropod and vertebrate cells. After being injected by the mosquito, the virus begins to multiply, but the immune system usually mobilizes its defenses to destroy the invader. However, in one case in every 200 to 300, the virus evades the defensive response and invades the human host, causing an often fatal illness.

THE ILLNESS

Five to fifteen days after the insect bite, the patients starts having flulike symptoms. Headache, fever, nausea, and vomiting are followed by confusion, restlessness, and difficulty speaking. Facial paralysis and Parkinson's-like "extrapyramidal" symptoms, including tremor, stiffness, and choreoathetoid (weird, twisting) movements, occur. The patient is rigid and reflexes are overactive. Convulsions are common, occurring in over 75 percent of pediatric patients. Blood tests specific for JE become positive in about four days. Until then, making the diagnosis depends on the history of exposure to mosquitoes during a transmission time, blood counts, CT scans or MRIs, and signs of diffuse brain inflammation. As the disease continues, its victim gradually falls into a coma. Death can be delayed and sometimes even prevented by life-support measures, which provide the time needed to begin recovery. Even with the best support, however, 30 percent of patients die. One-half of these survivors have permanent brain damage manifested by poor memory, behavioral problems, paralysis of a limb, or weakness and clumsiness.

TRANSMISSION

Cases occur primarily during a "transmission" period from March to October in tropical to semitopical areas and from May to September in cooler areas. JE is transmitted to man by Culex tritaeniorhynchus. This mosquito is zoophilic ("loves animals"), and we humans[2] are incidental innocent bystanders. From the virus's point of view, we are a dead end because the virus is in our blood only briefly, so we are not a good reservoir.

Only the female mosquito bites. The male has no need for food or anything else once his sexual mission has been accomplished. The female on the other hand needs the food to produce her eggs. A full blood meal takes two to seven days to digest, and she needs one to three meals in her life. In order to get a really good meal, when she bites, she injects her saliva, which contains the virus and an anticoagulant blood thinner. Her preferred entrée is pork, duck, or ardeid (wading) birds. In Far Eastern rural culture, contact between pigs and humans is fairly intimate, making the pig an excellent source of mosquito food as well as a virus reservoir. Birds are also a good choice for JE because they can widely disseminate the virions. Neither bird nor pig are made sick by JE, which amplifies its numbers with each transmission.

EPIDEMIOLOGY

Japanese encephalitis was first recognized in Japan in 1871, but the first major epidemic was described in 1924. There were more than 6,000 cases, with a frighteninig 60 percent mortality rate. Since then, JE has increasingly been recognized throughout most countries of Southeast Asia, where it is now the leading cause of viral encephalitis and where approximately 30,000 to 50,000 cases are reported each year. In endemic countries the disease primarily affects children under fifteen years of age. The World Health Organization reported 15,000 deaths from JE worldwide in 2001, with a fatality rate in symptomatic cases of between 5 and 35 percent. The available figures are underestimates because of underreporting and underdiagnosing.

In the second half of the twentieth century there were yearly outbreaks in the more temperate parts of Asia, including Japan, Korea, and parts of China. Japan experienced summer epidemics as late as 1966. Korea had a major epidemic in 1940, involving 5,616 cases, including 2,729 fatalities. Yearly epidemics continued, but 1958 was a terrible year for Korea, with 6,897 cases. Even so, the largest number of cases were in China. Between 1965 and 1975, over a million cases were reported.

Beginning in the 1960s, there was a remarkable decrease in the number of cases due at least in part to universal vaccination programs. In industrialized Korea, Japan, and Taiwan, the disease has almost disappeared.[3] The decline mysteriously began before mass vaccination.[4] Of great concern is that, at the same time that there has been a dramatic decrease in the number of cases, the disease has been slyly spreading, having arrived in Australia in the last few years.

JE is still found in rural areas of Asia. Rice paddy farming provides, unfortunately, an almost perfect habitat for the mosquito. Add to that reliance on the pig for its many products, and one can see why JE is still a public health problem there. In 1999, fifty persons in Malaysia died of "the plague of the orient" (JE). This apparently caused a panic in that the government ordered soldiers to kill all 300,000 pigs in the area. Thousands of villagers abandoned their homes as the slaughter began.

Other attempts at control of JE have included zooprophylaxis, in which the vector is diverted from humans to cows or other animals the mosquito might prefer. In Singapore pig breeding is forbidden, and imported pigs are immediately quarantined. The pig industry has been centralized so that pig-human contact is minimized.

Another approach is to control the mosquito population. Pesticide use and a reduction in the amount of land used for cultivation and changes in farming techniques have had some success.

TRAVELERS AND EXPATRIATES

Anyone traveling to endemic areas should consider vaccination. The decision depends on individual considerations. Overall risk is low. Only bites by a carrier species can transmit; vector mosquitoes have a JE infection rate of less than 3 percent; JE infection causes serious illness in less than one per 200 cases. Do the math—the overall chance of getting JE from one bite is less than one in a million.

Individuals can take measures other than vaccination to decrease the risk of infection. Travel outside of a transmission period makes getting a mosquito bite less likely. DEET applied to exposed skin and even to clothes is effective. These mosquitoes are crepuscular, so one should be indoors at dawn and dusk.

THE VACCINES

There are three vaccines produced worldwide. One is derived from mouse brain and is the one in general use. The other two, derived from golden-haired hamsters' kidney cells, are manufactured and sold only in China.

The sole available vaccine is derived from JE-infected mouse brain. The vaccine was licensed in the USA in the 1930s. At about the same time, Russia and Japan produced a mouse brain–based JE vaccine, but it was abandoned. In the forties our military prepared a rather crude formalin-killed vaccine that consisted of filtering the mouse brain extract and adding thimerosal. In the laboratory its immunogenicity was unpredictable, and the vaccine was never field-tested.

The current vaccine is a highly purified mouse brain extract. Putting neurological tissue in a vaccine is always a worry because it may possibly cause severe allergic reactions. Other concerns are contamination with unknown viruses (or prions!). The purification process is meant to remove any trace of neurological tissue. The extract undergoes ultracentrifugation, then ultrafiltration, protamine sulfate precipitation, and formalin inactivation in the cold followed by repeat ultrafiltration and ammonium sulfate precipitation. The vaccine is diluted as necessary to meet Japanese national standards and buffered with phosphate, then stabilized with gelatin and sodium glutamate and sterilized with thimerosal. The mouse brain vaccine is 100 percent effective in stimulating adequate antibody levels, but levels fall off quickly, so a three-dose schedule has been adopted in Japan.

TOXICITY

Of those vaccinated, 10 to 20 percent have pain and inflammation at the injection site. Chills, fever, nausea, vomiting, and abdominal pain occur in 10 percent. In 1945, 35,000 American soldiers on Okinawa received a crude mouse brain vaccine. Eight of the soldiers developed neuritis, but there was insufficient evidence to determine if the vaccine was the cause. One serviceman died suddenly sixty hours after vaccination.

Since 1989 a new kind of reaction has been seen. The patient develops hives, wheezing, and on occasion shock, requiring hospital treatment. The reaction appears to be related to certain lots of vaccine. This is still under investigation. In the meantime, persons who have a history of asthma or anaphylaxis should avoid the vaccine. The reaction occurred as long as two weeks after the shot.

Of great concern, a Danish study that reviewed the side effects of all patients between 1983 and 1989 indicated as many as one episode of encephalitis per 50,000 doses. This was a retrospective epidemiologic review and at variance with all other studies. A controlled prospective study has been called for. In Korea, public opposition to the JE vaccine has become intense. Since there have been virtually no natural JE cases in years, the vaccine is perceived as being more dangerous than the disease.

CONCLUSION

Although almost unknown in the West, JE has been a major public health problem in Asia. In the last thirty years the number of cases has decreased dramatically. The JE vaccine is undoubtedly an important element, but it should be noticed that the decline began long before routine immunization. Furthermore, there has been a decline even in unvaccinated communities. This decline is due to disruption of the pig-mosquito-bird cycle by urbanization, insecticides, and less reliance on rice paddy farming. Children in endemic areas should have boosters to maintain adequate antibodies until age ten.

Americans traveling to Asia do not need to be vaccinated for JE unless they expect to be in one of the high-risk categories.

CHAPTER 23

Rabies Vaccine

BACKGROUND

Rabies has been recognized and feared for thousands of years. The writers of ancient Mesopotamia, China, Greece, Rome, and India documented the awful progress of the disease.

> The patient can neither stand nor lie down, like a mad man; he flings himself hither and thither, tears his flesh with his hands, and feels intolerable thirst. This is the most distressing symptom, for he so shrinks from water and all liquids that he would rather die than drink or be brought near to water. It is then they bite other persons, foam at the mouth, their eyes look twisted, and finally they are exhausted and painfully breathe their last. (Girolamo Fracastoro, 1546)

Rabies occurs in warm-blooded animals all over the globe except in Australia, the U.K., and Antarctica. It is caused by a virus that attacks the brain; it is always fatal.[1] In the USA there have been one or two cases each year for the past decade. The disease is transmitted to humans by contact with an infected animal.

THE VIRUS

The virus has a strange life. Rabied animals, which carry the virus in their salivary glands, infect their victims by biting them. The virus remains quiescent at the bite site for a time, but sooner or later symptoms appear. The interval between bite and symptoms varies tremendously—from a few days to more than a year. The duration of this incubation period is affected by the number and depth of the bites and by their location on the victim. Bites on the head, face, or neck have shorter incubation times than do bites on the legs or hands.

Eventually the virus finds its way to a nerve and slowly follows it to its origin in the brain. As the infection spreads through the brain, the virus begins to travel in the nerves back from the brain to all parts of the body, including the salivary glands. The now rabid victim is ready to spread the infection to the next unfortunate animal it encounters. And so the cycle is completed.

THE ILLNESS

Symptoms begin with a mild flulike illness. The area of the bite may become painful or numb. During the ensuing week, symptoms increase and the patient has a fever. By this time the patient is already doomed. The victim begins having difficulty speaking, becomes disoriented, and is some-times agitated and aggressive. The patient develops seizures, muscle spasms, hallucinations, and massive whole-body response to noise, lights, and especially water. The victim has intense thirst but, diabolically, swallowing becomes agonizing and water, or even the thought of water, precipitates intense throat spasms. This living hell is called hydrophobia.

Dogs in this phase typify the mad dog, foaming at the mouth and attacking anything in its path. This has been described as furious rabies. In distinction, some humans move quickly on to the paralytic form, in which they experience lethargy, paralysis, and difficulty breathing. Without life support, which is pointless, death comes within two weeks.

EPIDEMIOLOGY

Worldwide, over 90 percent of human cases of rabies are due to bites by unvaccinated dogs. In rural areas, small animals, especially bats, are the predominant offenders. Oddly enough, the same is true for those cities that do have effective immunization programs for dogs. In cities that do not immunize, almost all cases are due to dog bites.

All warm-blooded mammals can get rabies but have different degrees of susceptibility. Foxes, coyotes, jackals, and wolves are most susceptible to rabies. Skunks, raccoons, bats, ferrets, and cattle are highly susceptible. Dogs, sheep, goats, horses, and subhuman primates are moderately susceptible. Opossums are considered a low risk for rabies because they are relatively resistant to the virus. Rodents (squirrels, rats, mice, and chip-munks) and rabbits are at low risk of becoming infected.

In the USA there have been only one or two cases per year since a strong dog and cat vaccination program was started in 1940s and '50s Most cases occur in young boys, in the summer, in rural areas. The most common transmitter of rabies in the USA is a strange creature known as the silver-haired bat (*Lasionycteris noctivagans*).

Any animal behaving strangely should be avoided. The rabied animal may appear to be friendly or hurt. Don't touch. Call the appropriate agency or the police.

Not all cases of human rabies are associated with a known bite. Bites of a sleeping victim may go unnoticed, but some cases appear to be due to nonbite contact. Contact with bat saliva droplets, especially on breaks in the skin or mucous membranes, may transmit the infection.

There have been cases of rabies among spelunkers who encountered dense masses of bat excreta. In these cases the illness may have been due to inhaled virus.

There have been six reported cases of transmission from person to person by corneal transplant. But in every series of cases, there are some that defy explanation.

TREATMENT AND PREVENTION

In the eighth century, a Dutch nobleman, Hubert, led a life of de-bauchery until, on a hunt, he saw a stag with a crucifix in his antlers, warning him to change his ways. Saint Hubert immediately gave away his possessions and became a monk. He later became patron saint of forest workers, hunters, opticians, metalworkers, dogs, mad dogs, and hydro-phobia. Pilgrims traveled great distances to Liege in the hope of finding a miracle cure. Saint Hubert's method was to brand the bite wound with a hot iron cross (key). In early cases of superficial bites, this cauterization may in fact have killed the virus, "miraculously" curing the petitioner. We have yet to do better. Pilgrimages to Liege continued through the nine-teenth century.

A different pilgrimage was going on in Louis Pasteur's laboratories. He and the band of brilliant scientists he gathered around him were changing the heart and face of science. Relics and miracles were giv-ing way to microscopes and petri dishes.[2] One of the "miracles" was the development of a rabies vaccine. Pasteur described his method in detail:

A dog may be rendered refractory to rabies in a relatively short time in the following way: Every day morsels of fresh infective spinal cord from a rabbit which has died of rabies, developed after an incubation period of seven days, are suspended in a series of flasks, the air in which is kept dry by placing fragments of potash at the bottom of the flask. Every day also a dog is inoculated under the skin with a Pravaz' syringe full of sterilized broth, in which a small fragment of one of the spinal cords has been broken up, commencing with a spinal cord far enough removed in order of time from the day of the operation to render it certain that the cord was not at all virulent. (This date had been ascertained by previous experiments). On the following days the same operation is performed with more recent cords, separated from each other by an interval of two days, until at last a very virulent cord, which has only been in the flask for two days, is used. The dog has now been rendered refractory to rabies.

Joseph Meister, aged 9 years, also bitten on July 4th, at eight o'clock in the morning, by the same dog. This child had been knocked over by the dog and presented numerous bites, on the hands, legs, and thighs, some of them so deep as to render walking difficult. The principal bites had been cauterized at eight o'clock in the evening of July 4th, only twelve hours after the accident, with phonic acid, by Dr. Weber, of Ville.

At the examination of the dog, after its death by the hand of its master, the stomach was found full of hay, straw, and scraps of wood. The dog was certainly rabid. Joseph Meister had been pulled out from under him covered with foam and blood.

The death of this child appearing to be inevitable, I decided, not without lively and sore anxiety, as may well be believed, to try upon Joseph Meister the method, which I had found constantly successful with dogs...

Consequently, on July 6th, at 8 o'clock in the evening, sixty hours after the bites on July 4th, and in the presence of Drs. Vulpine and Rancher, young Meister was inoculated under a fold of skin raised in the right hypochondria, with half a Pravaz' syringeful of the spinal cord of a rabbit, which had died of rabies on June 21st. It had been preserved since then, that is to say, fifteen days, in a flask of dry air.

In the following days, fresh inoculations were made. I thus made thirteen inoculations, and prolonged the treatment to ten days. I shall say later on that a smaller number of inoculations would have been sufficient. But it will be understood how, in the first attempt, I would act with a very special circumspection...

On the last days, therefore, I had inoculated Joseph Meister with the most virulent virus of rabies, that, namely, of the dog, reinforced by passing a great number of times from rabbit to rabbit, a virus which produces rabies after seven days incubation in these animals, after eight or ten days in dogs...

Joseph Meister, therefore, has escaped, not only the rabies which would have been caused by the bites he received, but also the rabies with which I have inoculated him in order to test the immunity produced by the treatment, a rabies more virulent than ordinary canine rabies...(Gerald Geison, *The Private Science of Louis Pasteur*, 1995)

This vaccine was never in production. Results were inconsistent and some batches had live, pathogenic rabies virus. At least a dozen iterations have been developed. All those containing neurological tissue caused severe reactions. In 1956 a virus grown in mouse brain was more successful and is still used in South America. Another vaccine, derived from duck embryo, is much safer, but is a weak vaccine, requiring as many as twenty-three daily injections. This rabies vaccine is used all over the world.

The big breakthrough came in the sixties, when virologists learned how to grow the rabies virus in human cell culture. This eliminated all animal products and neurological tissues. The vaccine derived from human cell cultures is called HDCV (human diploid cell vaccine). The vaccine is derived from the soup in which the infected human cells grow. The virus is chemically inactivated (killed) and prepared for use by addition of human serum, an antibiotic, and preservatives. All the rabies vaccine used in the USA is made in Lyon, France (Pasteur Merieux-Connaught). It was licensed for use here in 1980. There are several other vaccines in use or in development. The goal is a less expensive, effective rabies vaccine that can be produced in the large quantities needed in the Third World.

HDCV appears to be highly effective. A placebo study or traditional clinical trial cannot be done for ethical reasons. The vaccine, however, was administered to volunteers in Iran who had been bitten by rabid dogs or wolves. Those properly immunized survived; there was not one case of rabies. About 1.5 million doses of HDCV have been administered successfully.

PRE-EXPOSURE AND POSTEXPOSURE VACCINATION

Pre-exposure vaccination refers to vaccination for high-risk persons who have not had exposure to rabies. Pre-exposure vaccination is recommended for veterinarians, animal handlers, speleologists, mail carriers, and laboratory workers. The recommended dose of HDCV is three doses over a three-week period. A booster is recommended after one year. The need for subsequent bosters should be individualized.

Postexposure vaccination refers to treatment after exposure to the rabies virus has occurred. Five doses are given in twenty-eight days. An essential feature of postexposure treatment is the administration of RIG (rabies immune globulin). The intended purpose of the RIG is to immediately supply protective antibodies, giving the recipient's body time to mount its own active defense. The first available RIG was derived from the blood of a hyperimmunized horse. Serum sickness was a common complication, and efficacy was unpredictable. Current RIG is derived from immunized humans (HRIG) and so does not cause serum sickness.

Understandably, many are vaccinated unnecessarily. No one wants to take a chance with rabies. But unecessary immunizations are expensive and do cause reactions. Some data are available to help decide when to use the vaccine.

If the animal is a dog, and it is available and can be quarantined, observe it for ten days. If it remains perfectly healthy,[3] it does not have rabies. If the animal has an up-to-date vaccination, it probably does not have rabies. But be sure it has been appropriately vaccinated; don't take the owner's word—see documentation. There must be at least two doses.

If there is no scratch, bite, or contact with mucous membranes, immunization is generally not necessary unless the animal is a bat. Have a very low threshold for contact with bats—exposure to rabies from a bat may go unnoticed. If a bat just flies through a window, get vaccinated. In the USA, bats are the most common transmitter of rabies. As we noted earlier, squirrels and rodents don't carry rabies.

CONCLUSION

Worldwide, 4 million people are vaccinated against rabies every year. In the U.S., 30,000 to 40,000 persons are vaccinated, many unnecessarily. Rabies cannot be eradicated because of its presence in so many species in so many places. There is no effective treatment of established disease. Control of the number of human cases depends on avoidance, immunization of animals, especially dogs, and prompt immunization when appropriate. The rabies vaccines are among the most dramatically successful, making it possible to control the incidence of a devastating disease.

CHAPTER 24

Vaccines of the Future

Future vaccines will be more effective and safer. Researchers, I believe, will find vaccines against the Big Three infections: malaria, tuberculosis, and AIDS.

CONVENTIONAL VACCINES

The perfect vaccine would be easy to administer, free of side effects, and provide lifelong specific immunity after one dose. Also, it would be inexpensive and abundant. Such a vaccine, of course, does not exist and never will. The vaccines licensed in the USA are based on the classic technology that originated in the Golden Age of Microbiology over a hundred years ago.

Traditional techniques include use of live vaccines, killed whole vaccines, or purified single-component vaccines prepared from fragments or toxins of the offending microbe. Live vaccines (measles, mumps, rubella, smallpox) cause an infection by an attenuated, harmless cousin of the disease-causing microbes. These vaccines are among the most effective and long-lasting, but persons with an impaired immune system may become overwhelmed by even the attenuated strain, thus becoming infected rather than protected.

A major worry about live, attenuated vaccines is the possibility that the attenuated strain may revert to virulence. This possibility can experimentally be eliminated by genetic engineering techniques. Today's vaccine-preventable pathogens are attenuated by various laboratory techniques[1] that may induce only a small change in the organism. In that case, reversion to the virulent form occurs readily. But genetic engineering can penetrate deep into the pathogen's genetic code and cause irreversible changes that make return to virulence impossible. Such a vaccine against cholera has been licensed.

The toxoid is another type of vaccine; it is directed against a toxin produced by some microbes, but not the microbe itself. Working with these toxins has been a difficult and dangerous business; many deaths have occurred. In the case of pertussis and other microbes, the whole genetic text has been unraveled. A close reading can identify the genes that produce the toxin. Altering these genes ensures a harmless toxin that is still strong enough to be an effective vaccine.

Killed whole organism vaccines (pertussis, polio,[2] flu) cannot become virulent, but they may require boosters in order to maintain protection and commonly have side effects due to the smorgasbord of components of a whole organism.

Single-component or "purified" vaccines contain one or more specific components of the microbe-causing disease. These vaccines may be less effective than whole organism vaccines, but are still capable of causing severe reactions.

RECOMBINANT VIRAL VECTORS

Some of the problems associated with conventional vaccines may be solved through a form of genetic engineering known as recombinant viral vectors.[3] This procedure ties an ordinary vaccine to a harmless virus. The virus spreads through the whole body, carrying the vaccine with it. The immune system, sensing the presence of a live foreign virus, mounts a strong immune response to both the carrier (vector) and the vaccine. The immune response is more like the reaction to a natural infection, compared to that of an injected vaccine that bypasses the immune defenses of the mucous membranes.

VACCINE ADMINISTRATION

No vaccine will work if it is not administered properly. All the common vaccines, except for oral polio, are administered by injection,[4] which is expensive,[5] can cause complications, and may make vaccination frightening. Injection also requires facilities and trained personnel. Some of the conventional vaccines have to be kept frozen, others are in powder form that must be dissolved in special diluents before administration. These are some of the obstacles to universal vaccination.

A novel approach to these problems is the incorporation of vaccine into food. Scientists have been able to bioengineer potatoes, tomatoes, bananas, and other edible plants to manufacture vaccines. Furthermore, food vaccines stimulate the immune defenses located in the lining of the intestines and respiratory tract; injections bypass this process. Because these vaccines are located inside the cell of the plant, they are protected from the digestive juices that destroy conventional vaccines. In view of the strong public resistance to even minimal genetic engineering of food plants, my guess is that it will be a long time before the world is ready for a food vaccine.

Other anticipated advances include packaging vaccines in biodegradable microspheres that will prolong exposure to the vaccine, eliminating the need for booster shots. We can also expect more combination vaccines, requiring fewer shots.

DNA VACCINES

Conventional vaccines contain some harmless component (usually a protein) of the offending microbe. The immune system reacts by forming antibodies that will protect against a future "real" infection. By contrast, in DNA vaccines, some genetic material from the microbe is inserted into the recipient's cells. This genetic material (gene) causes the cells to produce the vaccine. The immune system sees this as an extremely dangerous attack that looks like the "real thing." The immune response is swift and powerful, mobilizing all the necessary killer and other lymphocytes as well as antibodies. Compared to conventional vaccines, the immune response is more intense and longer-lasting.

DNA vaccines are administered by conventional injection or a needleless gene gun that shoots microscopic DNA-covered gold particles. The "naked DNA" response can be intensified by inserting it into a live, harmless virus that will deliver the DNA to all parts of the body.

New vaccines will, of course, have new side effects. If recipients integrate the DNA into their own genetic makeup, much could theoretically go wrong, including the development of cancer or autoimmune diseases.

VACCINES FOR CANCER PREVENTION

Some cancers caused by viruses can be prevented by appropriate vaccines. These include liver cancer (Hepatitis B virus), some oral cancers

(EBV virus), and cancer of the cervix (HPV-human pappillomavirus) vaccines. Other cancers caused by viruses may be preventable. These vaccines are like our old, standard, preventive vaccinations, unlike the new vaccines used to treat cancers that have already occurred.

THERAPEUTIC VACCINES

Traditionally, vaccines have been used to prevent infectious disease. But in recent years[6] scientists have been able to use the power of the immune system to treat cancer and other noninfectious diseases.

Mistakes in the production of DNA and RNA create cancer cells all the time. The immune system attacks and kills these deviants before they can run amok. Sometimes the immune system fails; cancer is the result. The immune system may fail because it is impaired, as with HIV, old age, chemotherapy, or other immune suppressants. The cancer sometimes evades even an intact immune system, if the cancer cells deviate from normal cells in only a minor way or hide their presence by keeping the telltale surface proteins deep within the cell. One mode is to shed large amounts of surface cancer protein so that the immune cells cannot find the real cancer cells.

Cancer immunotherapy strengthens the immune system so it is able to recognize and attack the cancer cells. There are many ways to do this. One of the more promising ways is to take the patient's dendritic white blood cells, sensitize them to the cancer, and then inject them into the patient in the hope that the dendritic cells's critical immune function will be enhanced. Another approach is to use a chemical produced by a mussel-like sea creature, the keyhole limpet. This protein binds to cancer cells and fuels the immune system at the same time. Yet another approach is to develop anticancer antibodies and connect those up with a strong immune booster (adjuvant).

Many scientists in labs around the world are carrying this work forward.

Other new areas of vaccine research involve those diseases that are caused by autoantibodies. In these cases, the immune system is hyperactive, and the goal of therapy is not to stimulate, but rather to soothe the immune system. The patient's immune system goes awry and attacks the patient with antibodies against the self. This research focuses on developing antibodies against those autoantibodies. The "anti-antibody" approach has seen some experimental success in preventing arthritis, diabetes, thyroid disease, lupus, multiple sclerosis, and other conditions.

CONCLUSION

As our understanding of the immune system deepens, we will learn how to make better vaccines. There is the potential here to save millions of lives. But learning always comes with mistakes. New vaccines, like all new therapies, often meet with initial enthusiasm and later face resistance when side-effect cases accumulate.

CHAPTER 25

HIV Vaccines

By [the year] 2010 there will be 25 million children orphaned because of AIDS. This is a human atrocity that women and men must contend with together—and without the help of a vaccine.[1]

INTRODUCTION

AIDS came into my professional life in 1985, about five years after the discovery of the HIV (human immunodeficiency virus). He was the head of the fashion-design program at the university. He was tall and imposing and spoke in stentorian tones. He was energetic and flamboyant. He wore a big black cape and walked like a conquering hero. I had seen him six months before, for an odd, lingering cough. Now he was transformed. Thin, weak, coughing, feverish. He lived 10 more days. If we had today's treatment, he would have lived for ten more years. His spirit never left him; he buffed his nails that last afternoon.

There is of course no workable HIV vaccine. Many laboratories in many countries are designing and testing a whole range of vaccines. There are many obstacles to overcome, but I do not share Richard Horton's pessimism. I believe our scientists have the tools, the intelligence, and even the money to give us a vaccine.

THE ILLNESS

There has much been written about the origin of AIDS.[2] The preponderance of evidence indicates that HIV was a gift to humankind from the African green monkey. It did *not* come from the polio vaccine.[3]

HIV is transmitted (as everyone in the world should know by now) by sexual contact, transfusions, and intravenous drug use (IDU). Days or weeks after infection, the patient experiences a rash, fever, swollen glands, and possibly meningitis. The symptoms are very much like those of infectious mononucleosis. These initial symptoms are evidence of the first major battle between HIV and the patient's immune system. As a rule the patient appears to recover, but in reality the HIV has merely retreated to the lymph glands, where it continues to multiply but is held in check by the patient's immune cells.

There is a group of patients whose illness never progresses beyond this stage. These "nonprogressors" may have a genetic variation of their immune system that keeps the virus in check.

It came as a surprise when scientists learned that in the usual case, the virus may be producing up to 10^8 virus particles[4] daily, even when the patient appears healthy. For a time the immune system keeps up with the virus. The infected person may continue to feel well except perhaps for some dermatological problem, swollen glands, or minor yeast infections. Eventually, however, the lymphocytes become exhausted and depleted.

At this point the patient may experience the direct effects of HIV infection, including brain and neurological injury, anemia, the dreaded "wasting syndrome," and dementia.

As the immune cell count slowly continues to decline, the patient falls victim to myriad organisms that caused no problem when the immune system was intact. In the early years of the epidemic, my practice was stood on its head. Pneumocystis pneumonia, once an exotic rarity, was becoming ordinary. The bizarre had become commonplace. After thirty years in practice, I was seeing conditions that I had never seen before: fungus infections of the brain, amoebae in the intestine, the purple or black Kaposi cancers almost anywhere in the body, histoplasmosis in the eye, even tropical spastic paralysis.

The powerful new antivirals have changed the picture. The "death sentence" of AIDS became a chronic disease. Sick patients began to feel well. HIV patients looked just like anyone else. Significant others rejoiced. Lectures on death and dying lost some of their popularity.[5] The medical staff looked less at the patient and more at the graphs of the T cells and other lymphocytes. The AIDS clinic shed its spiritual aura and became very busy.

THE VIRUS

Virology is a tough subject to master. Here's a random sentence from a famous textbook: "The immune response to recombinant HIV-1 gp 120 has also been under active investigation with use of adjuvants such as alum or incomplete Freund's adjuvant (IF) and newer adjuvant formulations such as water-in-oil emulsions with saponin derivative QS21, enterobacteria cell wall derivatives, or muramyl dipeptide derivatives."

Tough as it is, we will have to at least brush shoulders with virology if we are to understand the potential for an HIV vaccine.

Let us first consider the anatomy of an HIV virion. It is very small. Its small size led to its discovery. In 1892, Dmitri Iwanowski, a botanist at the St. Petersburg Academy of Science, reported on his experiments with tobacco mosaic disease. He found that passing crushed tobacco leaves through a Chamberlain unglazed porcelain filter removed the bacteria, as expected. The novel part of his discovery was that the bacteria-free filtrate was capable of transmitting the disease to other tobacco plants. Iwanowski attributed his findings to faulty filters or to a bacterium small enough to pass through the filter pores.

At about the same time, Martinis Beijerinck, a botanist working in the Netherlands, made the same observations as did Iwanowski. But unlike Iwanowski, he recognized that they were onto something new and important. He called the substance in the filtrate "contagium vivium fluidum." His discovery of a virus, an incredibly small infectious entity capable of reproducing and able to live only in a living cell, was just around the corner.

Whatever was killing the tobacco was small enough to pass through the ceramic filter. Discovery of such an agent was the beginning of virology. If it was particulate, it was too small to see with a light microscope, which can magnify only 1,000 times. One can only imagine the excitement created by the invention of the electron microscope in the first half of the twentieth century. It could magnify more than 100,000 times. And there it was: a virus, a bumpy little sphere.

The HIV virion is spherical. It has a protein coat and/or a fatty cover. The surface is covered with structures that look like mushrooms. The head of the mushroom is called GP120 (glycoprotein, size 120). GP120 is a major player in HIV infection. The stem of the mushroom is anchored to the coat. These structures, like an Egyptian pyramid, hide a chamber containing the riches. In the case of our virus, the riches are proteins, enzymes, including RNA and reverse transcriptase.

When the free virion is transmitted to a new victim, the virus seeks out particular cells (APCs) of the immune system throughout the body. These cells have structures on their surfaces that interlock with GP120. In this way, virus and immune cell become tightly attached and then fuse together. The virus's reverse transcriptase allows the viral RNA to take over the cell's "brain." After a period of latency, the cell begins to synthesize viral protein fragments, which are assembled into a new virion, which leaves the hapless cell still making more copies of the the virion.

This process, especially the reverse transcription, is prone to error, creating many variations.

IMMUNE RESPONSES

The ideal AIDS vaccine would prevent AIDS for life after a single oral dose. It would be inexpensive, readily available, and have no side effects. Now, back to the real world.

It might be possible to develop a vaccine that does not prevent infection but allows the infected person to remain well, similar to the condition of the nonprogressors. Such a vaccine would not prevent infection and might paradoxically increase infection by encouraging risky behavior.

The immune system produces antibodies to the GP120 site on the HIV virus. But the response is too little, too late. Neutralizing antibodies arise between two and six months after infection and are of limited range and relatively weak. This is all in part due to a heavy protein coat that protects the GP120 antigen from attack by the antibodies. Further, the GP120 tends to form in groups of three, which confuses the antibody-producing cells.

Antibody production is one response to HIV infection. Another response is activation of a variety of immune cells (see chapter 2). Cytotoxic T lymphocytes (CTL) are a major defense mechanism against viral infection. They can detect and destroy cells infected with HIV. CTLs exist in a variety of inherited types, accounting for some of the differences from patient to patient. Ultimately, however, neither antibodies nor immune leukocytes prevent progression of HIV infection. The exceptions are those intriguing individuals who do not become infected in spite of repeated exposures, and the nonprogressors.

THE VACCINES

There have been many attempts to produce a useful HIV vaccine. There are at least twenty vaccines in Phase 1 testing now. (Phase 1 studies a drug's safety in a few dozen to one hundred people. This phase is designed to see how the body responds to the drug, and how it is metabolized or excreted. Phase 1 studies usually take several months. Phase 2 trials test whether or not a drug produces the desired effect. Phase 2 trials may take up to several months and involve several hundred patients. Phase 3 studies further examine the effectiveness of the drug as well as how it compares to current treatments. Phase 3 trials may involve thousands of patients and take several years to complete.)

THE PROBLEMS

The HIV virus is notorious for its constantly changing configurations. This instability is due in part to the error-prone reverse transcription process and in part to the propensity of virions to share their DNA with each other. The rapid replication of the virus, which can produce up to 10^{10} virions per day, also facilitates variation.

There are nine different HIV-1 subtypes. Each would need its own vaccine. Researchers are working on such multivalent vaccines (several vaccine varieties in one). Another theoretical solution would be production of a "broad spectrum" vaccine.

An even more fundamental problem is that we do not know what kind of immune response would be protective. Some patients have lots of GP120 antibody that seems to accomplish nothing. Many scientists believe that cellular immunity, not antibodies, are critical in preventing disease. I have made frequent references to "immune cells" and white blood cells to avoid making the whole story too complex, but I can't get away with it any longer.

There are sentinel cells, including macrophages, dendritic cells, and scavengers, known collectively as antigen-presenting cells (APCs) under the skin and all over the body. They travel around in the blood and lymph fluids, stopping off for a gourmet visit to the liver or running up to the spleen for a checkup. When the APCs detect a foreign antigen, they engulf and destroy it. A portion of the foreign antigen (usually a protein) is "presented," mafia-style, to a T cell (CD4+). If the T cell decides to "take care" of the foreigner, he calls up all the immune defenses we have discussed throughout this volume.

The role of cellular immunity versus antibody immunity is not fully understood. Also unknown is how the immune mechanism of the mucous membranes resists penetration by the virus. Researchers assume that, if possible, it would be desirable for a vaccine to stimulate humoral, cellular, and mucosal immune responses.

VACCINE TYPES

Subunit vaccines are fragments of the HIV coat. The vaccine is a recombinant; that is, the active vaccine component is manufactured by

genetically engineered organisms. These vaccines produce humoral antibodies, but they have not been successful in preventing infection. Their
relative safety is a big plus. There are several of these vaccines in various
stages of investigation.

Live recombinant vaccines are genetically changed, harmless microbes
that have been trained to manufacture HIV antigens. Since the vaccine is
live, cellular and mucosal immunity is stimulated. As we have seen,
however, live virus vaccines have a way of attacking a host who has an
impaired immune system or reverting to the virulent form.

Killed whole vaccines have been used for many infections. In the case
of HIV, the usual fear of possible reversion to a virulent form is especially
dangerous. There is concern that the killing process will decrease its an-
tigenicity. There is a Phase 3 study of such a vaccine in progress. DNA
vaccines, combinations of vaccines, pseudovirion, and "pox" vaccines are
other new modalities under study.

ETHICAL ISSUES

Clinical research always has some tension arising from overt or, more
often, covert ethical conflicts. Even in the most relaxed clinical study, in
which the patient knows and trusts the investigator and the feelings are
mutual, the tension is there. Even when the stakes are low, as in a clinical
study comparing two mild painkillers, the subject[6] and investigator have
different agendas. The patient hopes the study will provide relief and is
pleased to help the doctor's research. Free medication samples would be a
nice extra. The investigator hopes that he is able to recruit enough patients
to do a good clinical study and is pleased to comfort his patient. A mon-
etary bonus or journal article would be a nice extra.

Fast-forward now to a dusty African village where the white, English-
speaking investigator is trying to recruit a malnourished farmer to participate in an HIV vaccine program.

If informed consent is a problem in the first scenario, what is one to say
about the second one?

The Nuremberg Code was a reaction to the Nazi "medical" experiments
on humans. It is worth reading: Note numbers 1, 5, and 7 in particular.

THE NUREMBERG CODE

1. The voluntary consent of the human subject is absolutely essential.
   This means that the person involved should have legal capacity to

give consent; should be so situated as to be able to exercise free power of choice, without the intervention of any element of force, fraud, deceit, duress, over-reaching, or other ulterior form of constraint or coercion; and should have sufficient knowledge and comprehension of the elements of the subject matter involved as to enable him to make an understanding and enlightened decision. This latter element requires that before the acceptance of an affirmative decision by the experimental subject there should be made known to him the nature, duration, and purpose of the experiment; the method and means by which it is to be conducted; all inconveniences and hazards reasonable to be expected; and the effects upon his health or person which may possibly come from his participation in the experiment.

The duty and responsibility for ascertaining the quality of the consent rests upon each individual who initiates, directs or engages in the experiment. It is a personal duty and responsibility which may not be delegated to another with impunity.

2. The experiment should be such as to yield fruitful results for the good of society, unprocurable by other methods or means of study, and not random and unnecessary in nature.

3. The experiment should be so designed and based on the results of animal experimentation and a knowledge of the natural history of the disease or other problem under study that the anticipated results will justify the performance of the experiment.

4. The experiment should be so conducted as to avoid all unnecessary physical and mental suffering and injury.

5. No experiment should be conducted where there is an a priori reason to believe that death or disabling injury will occur; except, perhaps, in those experiments where the experimental physicians also serve as subjects.

6. The degree of risk to be taken should never exceed that determined by the humanitarian importance of the problem to be solved by the experiment.

7. Proper preparations should be made and adequate facilities provided to protect the experimental subject against even remote possibilities of injury, disability, or death.

8. The experiment should be conducted only by scientifically qualified persons. The highest degree of skill and care should be required through all stages of the experiment of those who conduct or engage in the experiment.

9. During the course of the experiment the human subject should be at liberty to bring the experiment to an end if he has reached the

physical or mental state where continuation of the experiment seems to him to be impossible.

10. During the course of the experiment the scientist in charge must be prepared to terminate the experiment at any stage, if he has probable cause to believe, in the exercise of the good faith, superior skill and careful judgment required of him that a continuation of the experiment is likely to result in injury, disability, or death to the experimental subject.

(Reprinted from *Trials of War Criminals before the Nuremberg Military Tribunals under Control Council Law No. 10*, Vol. 2, pp. 181–82. Washington, D.C.: U.S. Government Printing Office, 1949).

The obligation to protect experimental subjects from harm as further emphasized by the World Medical Association Declaration made at Helsinki in 1964. The declaration states that

The particular needs of the economically and medically disadvantaged must be recognized. Special attention is also required for those who cannot give or refuse consent for themselves, for those who may be subject to giving consent under duress, for those who will not benefit personally from the research and for those for whom the research is combined with care.

In any research on human beings, each potential subject must be adequately informed of the aims, methods, sources of funding, any possible conflicts of interest, institutional affiliations of the researcher, the anticipated benefits and potential risks of the study and the discomfort it may entail. The subject should be informed of the right to abstain from participation in the study.

Anyone who has been involved in clinical investigation as subject or investigator will immediately recognize the huge gap between the declarations and common practice.

One reason for this is that following these declarations to the letter would make many important clinical trials impossible. The documents make it clear—informed consent is the first principle of human experimentation. That kind of consent is impossible when the proposed study is based on concepts that are alien to the culture of the "volunteers" who enroll. I doubt that the creators of the Helsinki document imagined that the wealthy nations would be doing mass clinical trials in African nations.

The vaccine trials illustrate some of the ethical issues. Many researchers believe that even if a vaccine does not completely prevent infection, it may slow or even halt progression. The vaccine may allow the patient to feel well for a long time. Testing for this possibility should be simple and straightforward[7]—recruit a sufficient number of volunteers and give some the vaccine and some a placebo; over time it will be apparent if the vaccines prevent infection altogether or slow progression or do nothing. But there are problems with this. The investigator is morally bound to provide the best medical care for all the study subjects; the study may not deny the subject the benefit of any existing treatment, which in this case would mean providing anti-AIDS medication.[8] Here comes the dilemma: The anti-AIDS medication may mask the benefit of the vaccine. Millions of lives may be at stake. So, what do we do? Such questions have given rise to some strange conversations. What does the "best medical care" mean? Suppose the host country does not have the medication available. Does that mean that no care is the best care? Or does "best care" mean the best care possible in the host country? Or does it mean the best care in the world?

Most clinical trials of HIV vaccines are conducted in Africa by American researchers. Several circumstances make research in developing countries attractive. First, trials need a population with many HIV-infected persons.[9] Second, research in Africa is easier because there are fewer regulations and constraints, and in some ways the subjects are "a captive audience." Does this make it all right to conduct experiments that would not be allowed in the USA? Is it okay to study issues of potential benefit to the experimenters without regard for the needs of the host country, or to study treatments that the host country will not be able to afford? Additional incentives to do studies in Africa include lower risk of litigation, and populations willing to enroll in any study that seems to offer promise of medical help.

Conclusion

Although they had no word for it, the ancients knew that if you survived an infection, you would not catch it again: You were immune. The immune system is beautiful, but you cannot touch, feel, see, or smell it. It is everywhere. It consists of billions of cells that use chemicals as messengers to communicate with each other. It is more like a computer program than a machine.

If an infectious agent attempts to penetrate us, the frontline cells send out the emergency e-mail; killer cells rush to the scene, T cells display mug shots of the attacker's antigens so that the plasma cells can start producing custom-made antibodies, and soon a huge crowd of bystanders appears, creating pus, inflammation, and swelling. When the battle is over, assuming that you have won, the immune system will have changed. The memory cells roving through your body now know what the enemy looks like, and should it try anything funny, the immune system will be ready.

In the prevaccine era, every family lost a child or knew of one so lost due to vaccine-preventable diseases. Today in the USA, the death of a child is an unexpected tragedy; in the past it was an expected sorrow. Everyone knows about the miracle of vaccines. Smallpox, gone; polio and measles not far behind; in the USA, no polio, no measles, no congenital rubella syndrome, no diphtheria, no tetanus. The "big three" (AIDS, malaria, tuberculosis) still defy attempts to control them with vaccines, but this generation may yet see success.

Fooling the immune system can be difficult and dangerous. A serious error is to suppose that all vaccines are much the same. Vaccines are not all the same. Not at all. Some come from the exudate of a cowpox pustule, other are created through genetic engineering. Some are live viruses that infect the person being vaccinated. Sometimes the vaccinated person can infect others with the vaccine virus. Some vaccines are killed viruses or bacteria, other are made from purified components.

The same vaccines are not the same. The whooping cough vaccine until recently was made from whole bacterial cells. Now an "acellalar" vaccine that has much-reduced toxicity is available to those who can afford it. Mercury-free vaccines have been developed or are in the pipeline. A new variation of the Hib vaccine protects newborns for the first time. Sometimes manufacturers, for reasons of their own, change the formulation or composition of the vaccines they make. There are eleven different mumps vaccines made differently by different manufacturers.

The way you react to a vaccine depends on many factors, including your genes, previous infections and immunizations, and your general health. The same vaccine will be totally ignored immunologically by one individual, but create immunologic chaos in another. The very young and very old react differently.

Every vaccine has a history—none appears full-blown. Today we have just a glimmering of understanding of the immune system. Creation of a new vaccine necessarily requires animal experiments, clinical trials, and widespread use. There is no substitute, in the end, for experimentation on humans. No matter how careful and meticulous the experimentation, things sometimes go wrong. Every new vaccine brings new toxicities. The scientists manipulating the genes of pathogens are exploring the essence of life, and I can only wonder what new wonders and new griefs they will find. Every vaccine I know of has had false starts, unexpected toxicity, or unexplained failures. In some contexts a good vaccine can have a bad effect (see rubella, chapter 12). As I have documented, many children have died traveling the road to freedom from infectious disease.

There are obstacles inherent in the science. But the field of vaccinology has special societal obstacles: fear of the unknown, mandatory vaccination, a highly litigious environment, bureaucracy, self-serving politization, political turf wars, an all-powerful pharmaceutical industry, and irrational policy decisions. I take some comfort that there have been such problems since the first cowpox vaccine, but progress has continued nonetheless. A new world of genetically engineered vaccines is coming.

Finally, I must touch on some questions that have made me uncomfortable while doing the research for this book. How come most of the vaccines we do have are to protect against the diseases of the richer nations? How come there is a vaccine for chicken pox but none for malaria? How come infectious disease in the Third World ravages children who die by the millions of diseases preventable with today's vaccines? Let those with the energy to oppose vaccination turn their eyes to a wider world.

APPENDIX A

Recommendations

Recommended Childhood and Adolescent Immunization Schedule
United States · July–December 2004

Range of Recommended Ages | Catch-up Immunization | Preadolescent Assessment

Vaccine ▼ / Age ►	Birth	1 mo	2 mo	4 mo	6 mo	12 mo	15 mo	18 mo	24 mo	4-6 y	11-12 y	13-18 y
Hepatitis B[1]	HepB #1 (only if mother HBsAg (-))	HepB #2	HepB #2		HepB #3 →						HepB series	
Diphtheria, Tetanus, Pertussis[2]			DTaP	DTaP	DTaP		DTaP →			DTaP	Td	Td
Haemophilus influenzae Type b[3]			Hib	Hib	Hib	Hib →						
Inactivated Poliovirus[4]			IPV	IPV	IPV →					IPV		
Measles, Mumps, Rubella[4]						MMR #1 →				MMR #2	MMR #2	
Varicella[5]						Varicella →					Varicella	
Pneumococcal[6]			PCV	PCV	PCV	PCV →			PCV	PPV		
Influenza[7]					Influenza (Yearly) →	Influenza (Yearly) →				Influenza (Yearly)		
Hepatitis A[8]									Hepatitis A Series →			

Vaccines below red line are for selected populations

This schedule indicates the recommended ages for routine administration of currently licensed childhood vaccines, as of April 1, 2004, for children through age 18 years. Any dose not given at the recommended age should be given at any subsequent visit when indicated and feasible. ▨ Indicates age groups that warrant special effort to administer those vaccines not previously given. Additional vaccines may be licensed and recommended during the year. Licensed combination vaccines may be used whenever any components of the combination are indicated and the vaccine's other components are not contraindicated. Providers should consult the manufacturers' package inserts for detailed recommendations. Clinically significant adverse events that follow immunization should be reported to the Vaccine Adverse Event Reporting System (VAERS). Guidance about how to obtain and complete a VAERS form can be found on the Internet: www.vaers.org or by calling 800-822-7967.

1. Hepatitis B (HepB) vaccine. All infants should receive the first dose of hepatitis B vaccine soon after birth and before hospital discharge; the first dose may also be given by age 2 months if the infant's mother is hepatitis B surface antigen (HBsAg) negative. Only monovalent HepB can be used for the birth dose. Monovalent or combination vaccine containing HepB may be used to complete the series. Four doses of vaccine may be administered when a birth dose is given. The second dose should be given at least 4 weeks after the first dose, except for combination vaccines which cannot be administered before age 6 weeks. The third dose should be given at least 16 weeks after the first dose and at least 8 weeks after the second dose. The last dose in the vaccination series (third or fourth dose) should not be administered before age 24 weeks.

Infants born to HBsAg-positive mothers should receive HepB and 0.5 mL of Hepatitis B Immune Globulin (HBIG) within 12 hours of birth at separate sites. The second dose is recommended at age 1–2 months. The last dose in the immunization series should not be administered before age 24 weeks. These infants should be tested for HBsAg and antibody to HBsAg (anti-HBs) at age 9–15 months.

Infants born to mothers whose HBsAg status is unknown should receive the first dose of the HepB series within 12 hours of birth. Maternal blood should be drawn as soon as possible to determine the mother's HBsAg status; if the HBsAg test is positive, the infant should receive HBIG as soon as possible (no later than age 1 week). The second dose is recommended at age 1–2 months. The last dose in the immunization series should not be administered before age 24 weeks.

2. Diphtheria and tetanus toxoids and acellular pertussis (DTaP) vaccine. The fourth dose of DTaP may be administered as early as age 12 months, provided 6 months have elapsed since the third dose and the child is unlikely to return at age 15–18 months. The final dose in the series should be given at age ≥4 years. **Tetanus and diphtheria toxoids (Td)** is recommended at age 11–12 years if at least 5 years have elapsed since the last dose of tetanus and diphtheria toxoid-containing vaccine. Subsequent routine Td boosters are recommended every 10 years.

3. _Haemophilus influenzae_ type b (Hib) conjugate vaccine. Three Hib conjugate vaccines are licensed for infant use. If PRP-OMP (PedvaxHIB or ComVax [Merck]) is administered at ages 2 and 4 months, a dose at age 6 months is not required. DTaP/Hib combination products should not be used for primary immunization in infants at ages 2, 4 or 6 months but can be used as boosters following any Hib vaccine. The final dose in the series should be given at age ≥12 months.

4. Measles, mumps, and rubella vaccine (MMR). The second dose of MMR is recommended routinely at age 4–6 years but may be administered during any visit, provided at least 4 weeks have elapsed since the first dose and both doses are administered beginning at or after age 12 months. Those who have not previously received the second dose should complete the schedule by the visit at age 11–12 years.

5. Varicella vaccine. Varicella vaccine is recommended at any visit at or after age 12 months for susceptible children (i.e., those who lack a reliable history of chickenpox). Susceptible persons age ≥13 years should receive 2 doses, given at least 4 weeks apart.

6. Pneumococcal vaccine. The heptavalent **pneumococcal conjugate vaccine (PCV)** is recommended for all children age 2–23 months. It is also recommended for certain children age 24–59 months. The final dose in the series should be given at age >12 months. **Pneumococcal polysaccharide vaccine (PPV)** is recommended in addition to PCV for certain high-risk groups. See *MMWR* 2000;49(RR-9):1-35.

7. Influenza vaccine. Influenza vaccine is recommended annually for children aged ≥6 months with certain risk factors (including but not limited to asthma, cardiac disease, sickle cell disease, HIV, and diabetes), healthcare workers, and other persons (including household members) in close contact with persons in groups at high risk (see *MMWR* 2004;53:[RR-6]:1-40) and can be administered to all others wishing to obtain immunity. In addition, healthy children aged 6–23 months and close contacts of healthy children aged 0–23 months are recommended to receive influenza vaccine, because children in this age group are at substantially increased risk for influenza-related hospitalizations. For healthy persons aged 5–49 years, the intranasally administered live, attenuated influenza vaccine (LAIV) is an acceptable alternative to the intramuscular trivalent inactivated influenza vaccine (TIV). See *MMWR* 2004;53[RR-6];1-40. Children receiving TIV should be administered a dosage appropriate for their age (0.25 mL if 6–35 months or 0.5 mL if ≥3 years). Children aged ≤8 years who are receiving influenza vaccine for the first time should receive 2 doses (separated by at least 4 weeks for TIV and at least 6 weeks for LAIV).

8. Hepatitis A vaccine. Hepatitis A vaccine is recommended for children and adolescents in selected states and regions and for certain high-risk groups; consult your local public health authority. Children and adolescents in these states, regions, and high-risk groups who have not been immunized against hepatitis A can begin the hepatitis A immunization series during any visit. The 2 doses in the series should be administered at least 6 months apart. See *MMWR* 1999;48(RR-12):1-37.

For additional information about vaccines, including precautions and contraindications for immunization and vaccine shortages, please visit the National Immunization Program Web site at www.cdc.gov/nip/ or call the National Immunization Information Hotline at 800-232-2522 (English) or 800-232-0233 (Spanish). **Approved by the Advisory Committee on Immunization Practices (www.cdc.gov/nip/acip), the American Academy of Pediatrics (www.aap.org), and the American Academy of Family Physicians (www.aafp.org).**

APPENDIX B

Legal Aspects of Vaccination

Compulsory vaccination raises a tangle of emotional, legal, ethical, religious, medical, and political issues. We can begin the story with a Massachusetts law drafted in 1855 that allowed cities and other jurisdictions to require that children be vaccinated against smallpox in order to attend public school. Although there was evidence that this policy was of some efficacy in preventing smallpox, there was nonetheless an epidemic in Cambridge in May 1901. The Boston Health Department conducted an aggressive and effective vaccination program that brought the epidemic under control. Health workers visited work sites and even went from house to house in an attempt to vaccinate the whole population.

Persons who refused vaccination were subject to a five-dollar fine or fifteen days in jail. The Reverend Henning Jacobson, a courageous and energetic clergyman, defied the government and refused to be vaccinated. He was duly prosecuted, and the case ultimately made its way to the U.S. Supreme Court. Justice Harlan wrote in part:

> The defendant insists that his liberty is invaded when the state subjects him to fine or imprisonment for neglecting or refusing to submit to vaccination; that a compulsory vaccination law is unreasonable, arbitrary, and oppressive, and, therefore, hostile to the inherent right of every freeman to care for his own body and health in such way as to him seems best; and that the execution of such a law against one who objects to vaccination, no matter for what reason, is nothing short of an assault upon his person. But the liberty secured by the Constitution of the United States to every person within its jurisdiction does not import an absolute right in each person to be, at all times and in all circumstances, wholly freed from

restraint. There are manifold restraints to which every person is necessarily subject for the common good.

This ruling has been the bedrock of precedence for forced vaccination. During epidemics and other health emergencies, the state acquires extraordinary powers, including incarceration. But even in the absence of an emergency, the courts have, in matters of health, consistently put the common good before individual rights.

This stance, however, runs afoul of a critical element of modern medical practice, namely patient autonomy and the absolute requirement of informed consent to any medical procedure. The package insert in all vaccines, textbooks, and law books states that an individual must be advised of any risks before consenting to a procedure. Consent, however, implies the possibility of dissent, of refusal. In the case of forced vaccination, we have informed nonconsent or, more often, uninformed nonconsent.

How is it possible for two such mutually exclusive concepts to exist side by side? Vaccination has become a part of U.S. culture; "getting shots" is an accepted rite of passage. Additionally, there are exemptions from vaccinations. All states have medical exemptions. If a qualified practitioner certifies that a child should not receive one or more vaccines for medical reasons,[1] an exemption may be made.

Some states (less than one-third) also have religious or philosophical or "personal belief" exemptions. These exemptions are often very difficult to obtain and require a brave parent and possibly a clergyman and lawyer. The court must be convinced that the individual or parent has a genuine, sincere religious objection to vaccination. If the exemption is denied and the parents try to defy the state mandate, their children may be excluded from school[2]; the parents may be charged with criminal child abuse or neglect, and the state may take custody of the children The intimidation and coercion are so intense that less than 2 percent of those who apply for an exemption obtain one.

The USA, known for its commitment to individual freedom and rights, takes an unusually aggressive stance with regard to vaccination. In the U.K., vaccination is voluntary, but their vaccine rates are comparable to ours.

Theoretically, the individual states control the compulsory vaccination programs. In some states the department of health decides vaccine policy; in other states, policy is legislated.[3] In both cases, however, there is tremendous pressure to follow federal guidelines. State health departments depend heavily on federal dollars, which may be withdrawn if the state does not meet federal quotas. The power and prestige of the CDC and other administrative heavy artillery easily intimidates state legislators and even health care professionals who might otherwise deviate from the official path.

There is a committee called the ACIP (Advisory Committee on Immunization Practices) established by federal statute that "shall provide advice and guidance to the...CDC regarding the most appropriate application of antigens [vaccines]...and recommend improvements in the national immunization efforts."

The ACIP sees its mission as encouraging vaccine usage. The CDC generally follows the "advice" of the ACIP about which vaccines to mandate. There are fifteen members on this powerful committee, all appointed by the secretary of Health and Human Services for their expertise in immunization. There are one or more members to represent consumers and community aspects of the programs. Finally, there are eight nonvoting ex officio members who represent the host of government health-related organizations.[4] These individuals often have ties to the pharmaceutical industry, and conflict of interest issues are so common that special exemptions have had to be provided. But this is where the critical decisions are made.

The "advice" of ACIP is what trickles down, with the force of law, to your doctor's office or clinic.

VACCINE LEGAL LIABILITY

As almost every other topic related to vaccines, the legal aspects are controversial, muddy, and constantly changing. A typical scenario would go like this: A healthy child becomes ill sometime after receiving a vaccination. The parents believe that the vaccine has caused the illness and file suit. The first question is: Did the vaccination cause the illness? If the answer is determined to be "yes," then liability revolves around a second set of questions.

- Was it appropriate to administer the vaccine with regard to patient age, allergy, prior reactions, seizures, or immunosuppression?
- Was the vaccine properly administered? Some vaccines must be kept frozen. Some must be injected under the skin, others into the muscle.
- Was the patient or guardian informed of possible side effects and reactions?

- Were adequate records kept? This includes type of vaccine, manufacturer, and batch and lot number.
- Was the vaccine properly manufactured and stored and free of defects or contamination?

If the answer is yes to all of the above, the courts have historically found in favor of the defendant pharmaceutical company. If the answer is no, the case is more likely to be won by the plaintiff.

The informed consent issue has some unique convolutions revolving around the question of who is responsible for informing the patient. Traditionally, the clinician administering the vaccine has been assigned that task. If you have ever read the package insert of any vaccine, you know that the list of possible adverse reactions is frightening. I think very few patients ever see that material, which often is an attempt by the manufacturer to disclaim any responsibility rather than provide information. In any case, the manufacturers have taken the position that it is up to the clinician to describe the vaccine risks. The courts have usually agreed with this view. As we noted, however, the clinicians do not provide comprehensive risk information because it would be time-consuming, would scare the patient, and in the end, the mandated vaccine is almost always administered.

A number of suits since 1974 changed the legal landscape. That year in *Reyes v. Wyeth Laboratories,* Wyeth was found liable for failure to inform a patient that its polio vaccine might cause polio. Wyeth sold the vaccine to the Texas Department of Public Health for distribution by the health department for a mass immunization campaign. The manufacturer's package insert contained appropriate warnings. The vaccine was distributed to the county health departments for administration. In the *Reyes* case the vaccine was administered by a nurse who did not inform the patient that there was a minute possibility of contracting polio from the vaccine. The court ruled that the manufacturer should have known that, under the conditions of a mass immunization program, it was likely that each patient would not be apprised of the risk and therefore Wyeth should have ensured that the patient would be informed. This decision against Wyeth was a kidney punch to the pharmaceutical industry.

Less than two years later, in 1976, epidemiologists predicted a severe swine flu epidemic. The government recommended a massive immunization program, which immediately became caught up in the presidential politics of the day.[5] Citing the *Reyes* decision and the dangers of using a new vaccine on a massive scale, the pharmaceutical industry balked at the production of the swine flu vaccine.[6] This prompted hasty legislation, which assigned vaccine liability to the federal government; affected individuals could sue the government, instead of the vaccine manufacturers, for damages. The epidemic never materialized, but the vaccine caused some cases of GBS paralysis, for which the government paid out more than $90 million in injury claims.

During the next decade these decisions encouraged frequent and costly litigation (sometimes in the millions of dollars) against the pharmaceutical manufacturers. Ironically, the success of vaccines increased the likelihood of litigation. Since the vaccines are administered to healthy children to protect them from diseases that neither the courts nor the plaintiff[7] had ever seen or experienced, the benefit is not obvious, but any adverse reaction at all is conspicuous and may be considered unacceptable. Furthermore, some state laws allowed children plaintiffs to sue for a predetermined period after they had reached adulthood. This effectively raised the statute of limitations by many years, increasing potential liability. Delayed litigation is complicated by loss of records, death of individuals, and failing memory of events ten or more years previous.

The pharmaceutical industry responded by withdrawing from the market. Manufacturers of DPT decreased from seven to two; oral polio vaccine from three to one; measles vaccine from six to one.

The entire vaccine program was in crisis. Intensifying pressure for some kind of fix was coming (each for their own reasons) from the public, medical organizations, federal health-related programs, trial lawyers, and pharmaceutical manufacturers. The result was the 1986 national childhood Vaccine Injury Compensation Program (VICP), which sought to facilitate compensation for vaccine injuries while at the same time limiting the cost of litigation and awards.

Compensation is facilitated by a no-fault process that is less formal and more rapid than conventional liability suits. The heart of the legislation is the "table" of known adverse effects. Any claim made that appears on the table is accepted at face value and results in an almost automatic award. The size of the award is based on the extent of the injury, as determined by a compensation board.

The cost of the program is controlled by caps on pain and suffering, lost wages, and attorney fees. There is no compensation for injuries claimed by any person other than the one who received the vaccination as, for example, in transmission of a live virus vaccine to a household contact. Under the act, a claim of vaccine injury must be submitted to the VICP before any other legal action. If the claimant does not accept the VICP award, they can then pursue other legal remedies, but they forfeit any further appeal to the board.

The act requires that all known or suspected adverse reactions be reported in order to monitor the toxicity of vaccines and make appropriate clinical and administrative changes. Unfortunately, many, indeed most, reactions are not reported by clinicians because of the work involved or failure to recognize that an adverse event has occurred.

Assessment of the efficacy of the act depends on who is doing the assessing, and when. The medical mainstream opinion seems to be that the act has achieved or approximated its main goals. Critics of course point to many problems with it. As we noted, the table is critical to success. When the act was formulated in 1986, it was based on the best information then available. As more vaccine-related data accumulated, the table required revision, which facilitated some claims (chronic arthritis due to German measles vaccine) but made others more difficult (seizures and shock due to DPT). These revisions have been contentious, and changes to the table have not been up-to-date; the last one was in 1994.

The processing of claims has at times been slower than anticipated. Twice in the early days of the act there was no money available for awards. It literally took an act of Congress to fund the program. Changes in the law have now put the program on a sound financial footing. An excise tax on pharmaceutical products has created an enormous fund sufficient to easily cover anticipated injury awards.

As old vaccines are improved and new ones are introduced, the liability picture will remain of great interest to the stakeholders.

APPENDIX C

Clinical Trials

INTRODUCTION

This information may help us evaluate the claims and counterclaims made by advocates and critics of various vaccines and other immunizations. Clinical trials when properly done are the scientific gold standard; they are the "proof" that a vaccine does or does not work. Sometimes it is impossible for practical reasons to do a formal clinical trial, and it becomes necessary to rely on epidemiological or historical data. Statistics are regularly used and abused in the analysis of these data. Let us explore some of these issues.

CLINICAL TRIALS

There are two critical questions about a vaccine or any other medical intervention: 1) Is it effective? 2) What are the adverse effects?[1] The scientific answer to these questions comes from *clinical trials*.

Suppose we want to see if a treatment that we have some reason to think might work really does work. The obvious clinical trial would be to give patients the treatment and see if they get better. If they do get better, we might be tempted to claim discovery of a new cure. But maybe the patients got better by themselves.[2] Or perhaps, in the case of prolonged treatment, our cure coincided with a change in season or improved sanitation or some other *confounder* that was the real cause of the improvement. To overcome these doubts we recruit a *control* group that does not receive the treatment. At the end of the trial we compare the control group that received no treatment with the *experimental* group that did receive the treatment. If the experimental group has fared better, we can claim that, based on our *controlled clinical trial*, our treatment is beneficial.

The control group is supposed to be just like the experimental group in all ways; the only difference between the groups is supposed to be whether or not they received the treatment. But there are many situations in which there are likely to be important differences between the control and experimental groups. Suppose, for example, that we want to do a controlled trial of a new vaccine. Suppose that we invite a group to volunteer for the trial, using those who agree as the experimental group and those who decline as the control group. There is a very good chance that the two groups will be quite different with regard to health consciousness, lifestyle, diet, exercise, perhaps smoking, and other confounders that might affect the likelihood of getting the infection that we are trying to prevent. A difference in the infection rate might be due to one of these or other, unknown, factors rather than the vaccine.

The way around this problem is to use only the volunteers and assign some of them to the experimental group and some to the control group. To avoid bias,[3] the assignments should be done randomly; there are computer programs that can randomly select members from a given list. There may be some difficulty recruiting volunteers when they are informed that on the toss of a coin, so to speak, they will or will not receive the vaccine. But once we do have the volunteers and they are assigned to the experimental or control groups, we have a *randomized, controlled clinical trial*.

But what about the placebo effect? Placebo, from the Greek "to please," is an inert substance ("sugar pill") that has mysterious and powerful effects. The belief that the placebo is a "real" medication can affect blood pressure, heart rate, chest pain, bowel movements, and yes, even the immune system. So how do we know that the effect we see in the clinical trial is due to the vaccine rather than the powerful placebo effect of an injection supposedly containing a highly active biologic agent? The way around *this* problem is to give an injection of an inert substance, the placebo, to the control group. Of course the volunteers must not know if they are getting the placebo or the active vaccine. The subjects are said to be blinded in this regard. So now we have a *single blind randomized, controlled clinical trial*.

One more hurdle. If the doctors know who is getting the placebo and who is getting the vaccine, they are likely to treat the two differently. They may examine the experimental group more carefully, may question them more closely, may pay more attention to them. They may, if they believe in the treatment, also be more optimistic about the outcome for the experimental group. All this is communicated to the patient by the doctor's body language, enthusiasm, and affect. Even if the doctor tries very hard to be neutral, the unconscious, nonverbal message may come through. The solution? Blind the doctor. The doctor is not to know if the injection is the placebo or the active agent. We have arrived at the holy grail: *a prospective double blind randomized, controlled clinical trial.*

Of course there are many obstacles to the successful completion of such clinical trials. It is often impossible to maintain the blind. The vaccine may cause a sore arm; the blood count may be affected; patients have even been known to get their blood analyzed to see if they are taking the active agents or a placebo.[4] To get accurate results, sometimes hundreds of patients must be recruited and kept on protocol for years; such trials involve enormous costs and administrative headaches. And when the trial is finished and published in a medical journal, the fight over the interpretation of the results begins.

First to attack are the statisticians who point out that the statistical analysis was wrong: The chi square test was used instead of the Fisher two tail test. Next come the clinical investigators who point out that a faulty randomization method was used. Finally come the practitioners who point out that the results obtained under the carefully controlled condition of the trial cannot be duplicated in an office practice, where the patients often have multiple ailments, are already on conflicting medications, and are old and sick: all circumstances that were excluded from the clinical trial.

Another issue is the definition of success. Let me note here that the vaccines discussed in this book are the "conventional" vaccines designed to prevent various infections. There are "therapeutic" vaccines to treat individuals already infected; I will mention those only in passing. In the case of a conventional vaccine to prevent infection, the ideal end point would be, obviously, prevention of the infection. Like any treatment designed to prevent something, proof may be difficult since the goal is for nothing to happen, so how can you be sure that the treatment is working? In the case of vaccines, the gold standard of preventing infection will be especially hard to attain if the infection rate in the community is already low. To get around this obstacle, a surrogate end point may be used, such as serum antibody levels or the ability of the blood to kill the infectious agent in a test tube.

There are ethical issues, too. Since a clinical trial would be done only if there was some evidence that the proposed treatment might be effective, how can we justify giving half the patients a placebo? The answer is that it would be unethical NOT to prove or disprove the value of the treatment. The history of medicine is crowded with accounts of popular treatments (such as "bleeding," which probably finished off George Washington) that were widely accepted but actually harmful.

Young, brilliant Dr. Halsted developed the radical mastectomy more than a hundred years ago. The logic was irresistible: Cut away as much of the disease as possible—in this case the entire breast and the major muscles of the chest wall and all the lymph glands in the armpit. The results were dismal, but the less the surgery cured, the more radically it was pursued, culminating in the first half of the twentieth century in ultraradical mastectomies in which breast, muscles, lymph nodes, ribs, and even whole arms were removed. The cycle did not really end until a group of Italian surgeons, led by Dr. Varonesi of the Milan Tumour Institute, had the courage, in the 1980s, to do clinical trials comparing extensive surgery to conservative surgery plus radiation. Clinical trials showed that the century-old "accepted wisdom" was found wanting: The lesser surgery was better.

In the 1980s it was known that after a heart attack, certain types of rhythm irregularities of the heart were associated with sudden death. Encainide and other so-called antiarrhythmic drugs regulated the heartbeat and so were widely prescribed. But a placebo-controlled trial showed that the death rate of treated patients was actually higher than that of the placebo group, so much so that the clinical trial had to be ended prematurely.

This is an example of the importance of a placebo trial, and also shows how a surrogate end point (regularity of heart rhythm instead of mortality) can be misleading.

The ethical context gets stickier when a partially effective treatment is available, but the investigator wants to test a new treatment against a placebo. The placebo makes for better science, but patients may be unwilling to participate. This issue became acute during the early years of the HIV epidemic, when organized groups of patients aggressively opposed "death by placebo." It is now unusual to use a placebo when an accepted treatment already exists.

The ethics of human experimentation is an enormous topic far beyond the scope of this book, but we will touch on some issues later. For now I would just mention the circumstance in which clinical trials are conducted in Third World countries (or inner cities here) where there is no hope that the treatment will ever be available because of the cost. The charge is made that the poor are the guinea pigs while the wealthy benefit from the results of the clinical trial.

PERCENT OF WHAT?

Suppose there were three different vaccines for one infection. Suppose that the first vaccine reduced the infection rate by 50 percent, the second vaccine reduced the infection rate from 2 to 1 percent, and the third vaccine was such that one hundred patients would need to be treated to prevent one infection. Which vaccine is the best?

The answer of course is that all three are the same; it all depends on how you present the statistics. Studies have shown that even physicians, a supposedly sophisticated group, will be influenced by the manner in which the data are presented. The investigators who studied our hypothetical vaccine, and the pharmaceutical company manufacturing the vaccine, and the newspaper article about the vaccine will prefer to report a 50 percent reduction (known as the *relative risk reduction*) because it sounds better than the reduction from 2 percent to 1 percent (known as the *absolute risk reduction*), or the need to treat one hundred persons in order to prevent one infection *(number needed to treat; NNT)*.

The American Cancer Society frequently cites the statistic that 11 percent of women will develop breast cancer in their lifetime. This would be true if all women lived to age eighty-five. Since that is not true, and since breast cancer is more common in older women, the "statistic" is misleading. At age forty years, one woman in one thousand gets breast cancer each year.

In his marvelous book *Innumeracy*, John Allen Paulos (Vintage Books, 1988) cites this and the following examples of misleading data and statistics.

A newspaper headline screams "Holiday Carnage Kills 500 Over 4 Day Weekend"; but that is the usual number of deaths in any four-day period.

Suppose that you are informed that you have a condition that is associated with an average life span of only five years. It could mean that most people live five years; but it could also mean that some live many years while others succumb in weeks. Information about an "average" means little without some indication of the spread of values hidden in the average.

WHERE IS THE DENOMINATOR?

Some years ago it was noted that in one year there were twenty-eight teenage suicides among avid players of the Dungeon and Dragons computer games. This understandably caused much consternation and it was widely reported in the press. What was not mentioned was that there were 3 million players of the game that year. In this case knowing the denominator (3 million) changes the significance of the numerator (28). There may be a connection between the game and suicide, but if so it must be a rare event.

CORRELATION, COINCIDENCE, AND CAUSATION

It is reported that day care centers that ranked the best according to government criteria had the highest frequency of sexual abuse.

An epidemiologist notes that the overall cancer rate is lower in poor countries than in rich countries.

These are two examples of correlations or associations that are not cause and effect. In the day care example, further study shows that the good centers have better surveillance and more accurate reporting of the abuse, but actually have a lower frequency of it. In the cancer example, comparisons of individuals of the same age shows an opposite correlation—the poor have more cancer. But because the wealthy live longer and cancer is more common among the elderly, the cancer rate will be higher for that population.

A child develops fever and has a convulsion forty-eight hours after receiving a vaccine. Was this caused by the vaccine or is it a coincidence?

In trying to distinguish coincidence from causation, researchers look for specific clues. Ideally there are two distinct but similar groups, one exposed to the condition in question and one not exposed. In our vaccine example, we would look for a group of children who had received the vaccine and a group exactly the same but who had not had the vaccine. If the convulsion rate was the same in both groups, we would conclude that the vaccine did not cause the seizure. If the vaccinated group had more seizures, we would draw the opposite conclusion. In the real world, however, two such groups may be hard to find. If the vaccination rate is very high, there may not be enough nonvaccinated children for comparison. And if the nonvaccinated children belong to a special group that refuses vaccines, there may be other cultural and health differences that make them a noncomparable group.

Even if there are two groups, it is important to avoid or at least identify biases. The history of seizures must be obtained in the same way. The vaccine group may be questioned more closely or the parents may be more likely to remember that there was a seizure if it occurred near the time of the vaccination. Such differences may be misleading.

Has the problem cropped up in other groups, or in other locations and at other times? If reports come from the U.S., Brazil, and the Netherlands, we are more likely to take it seriously than if only one small group seems affected.

Is it certain that the vaccine definitely was given before the first seizure? The parents may not remember that the child had had a seizure before getting the vaccine, especially if they are convinced that the vaccine caused the seizure. Sometimes it is hard to tell which came first. A study done in a Veterans Administration hospital found that patients admitted with a heart attack were more likely to have been taking aspirin than patients without heart trouble, suggesting that aspirin caused the heart attacks. This counterintuitive observation was clarified when further study showed that the heart patients were taking aspirin because they had been having mild heart pains before the heart attack. The chest pain caused the aspirin-taking, not the other way around.

Another, obvious, clue is the strength of the association. If every child has a seizure, there will be little doubt about cause and effect. But if one in a thousand has a seizure, the issue will be much more difficult to judge.

If the reaction in question was unique and occurred only in vaccinated children, it would point to a cause-and-effect relationship. But if, as in the case of our seizure example, the reaction is common in nonvaccinated children, the connection becomes tenuous.

Does the association make sense? Large computer databases make possible what researchers disparagingly call data dredging. You can find all sorts of correlations, like coffee consumption and make of car, or marital status and odd or even house number. In the case of our hypothetical vaccine, a febrile convulsion is biologically plausible. Vaccines may cause fever and fever may cause seizures in susceptible children. If the vaccine administration correlated with thunderstorms, we would be most skeptical of cause and effect no matter what the statistics suggested.

STATISTICAL INSIGNIFICANCE

The eleven o'clock news anchorperson tells us that there is a new medicine for headaches, as reported in the ever-popular *New England Journal of Medicine*. The author of the article is quoted as saying that the studies of the new medicine showed a statistically significant effect on the intensity and duration of headaches. Sound good?

The medical literature is full of statistically significant effects. Statistically significant means that it is very unlikely that the effect being observed is due to chance. The effect may be small, even tiny, but it is still statistically significant. In the case of our hypothetical new headache remedy, it turns out that only 3 percent of patients get relief. But there is no doubt about it; 3 percent do get relief. The effect is statistically significant. But is it of practical significance? Maybe. But if the new medicine costs five dollars per tablet and causes heartburn in half the people who take it, we will say statistically significant, but clinically insignificant.

COSTS VERSUS BENEFITS

No matter how beneficial, every treatment, every drug, every vaccine has a cost. There is a direct dollar cost, and there may be indirect dollar costs such as loss of time from work, side effects, and toxicity. Other subtle costs include worry about the vaccine on the one hand and overconfidence in the vaccine's efficacy (which might result in careless behavior) on the other.

You do not truly understand an intervention unless you know both the costs and the benefits. Only then can you make a reasoned decision about the value of the intervention.

But advocates of a new vaccine focus only on the benefits, and opponents focus on the costs. In her book *Vaccination: The Issue of Our Times* (Mothering Magazine, Santa Fe, New Mexico, 1997), Peggy O'Mara writes "It is immoral to risk the health of even one child in order to save the lives of many." This is an extreme position that does not strike a reasonable balance between costs and benefits. Taken to its logical conclusion, this stance would exclude virtually all medical treatments. (There is a subtext here of the individual versus society.)

Patients sometimes see only the cost, as in the case of a woman who stopped taking her stroke-preventing medication because it made her mouth dry. It seems to me that in this case the benefit far outweighs the cost. But to her, the tangible cost of dry mouth and loss of taste outweighed the hypothetical benefit of avoiding a stroke at an unknown time in the future.

Sometimes the focus is all on the benefits, as in the case of taking a potentially toxic antibiotic for six months just to cure an ugly fungus infection of the toenail (which is likely to recur).

CONCLUSION

Every day we are exposed to opinions and statistics that are more about promoting a preconceived agenda than advancing science or reason. This is true in many areas of life, and medicine, and certainly in discussions of vaccines. Think about the numbers, and be skeptical.

Notes

Introduction

1. Tuberculosis from cows, anthrax from rabbits, pneumonia from parrots, swine flu from pigs, avian flu from birds, SARS from civet cat, avian flu from ducks, salmonella from turtles, HIV from nonhuman primates, BSE from cow brain, West Nile disease from birds, Ebola from the jungle, and rabies from bats are some examples.

2. The possibility of bioterrorism makes even the smallpox success contingent.

3. Even if one dose is expensive, most vaccines are given only once or twice in a lifetime—compare with medicines for chronic diseases like high cholesterol.

Chapter 2

1. Roy Porter, *The Greatest Benefit To Mankind* (New York: W. W. Norton, 1997), p. 275.

2. T. Vesikari and A. Z. Kaikian, "A Comparative Trial of Rhesus Monkey (RRV-1) and Bovine (RIT) Rotavirus Vaccines," *The Journal of Infectious Diseases*, 1986; 153(5):832–39.

3. T. H. Goh, "Resurgence of Mumps in Singapore Caused by the Rubini Mumps Virus Vaccine Strain," *The Lancet*, 1999; 354:1355–56.

4. L. A. Hanson, "Breast-feeding Provides Passive and Likely Long-Lasting Active Immunity," *Annals of Allergy, Asthma & Immunology*, 1999 May; 82(5):478.

5. N. A. Halsey, "Limiting Infant Expose to Thimerosal," *Journal of the American Medical Association*, 1999; 282(18):763–64.

6. P. Grandjean, P. Weihe et al., "Cognitive Performance of Children Prenatally Exposed To "Safe" Levels of Methylmercury," *Environmental Research*, 1998; 77(2):165–72.

7. See http://www.antigenics.com/whitepapers/qs21_adjuvant.html.

8. Alum is in DTP, pneumococcal conjugate, HIV, and hepatitis A vaccines.

Chapter 3

1. A. V. Richman et al., "Avian Leukosis Antibody Responses," *Proceedings of the Society for Experimental Biology and Medicine*, 1972; 139:235–37.

2. See http://www.vaccines.plus.com/B-EDDY-AND-TUSKAGEE.html/.

3. K. Shah and N. Nathanson, "Human Exposure To SV40: Review and Comment," *American Journal of Epidemiology*, 1976; 103:1–12.

4. O. P. Heinonen et al., "Immunization during Pregnancy against Poliomyelitis and Influenza in Relation to Childhood Malignancy," *International Journal of Epidemiology*, 1973; 2:227–235.

5. M. Carbone et al., "New Molecular and Epidemiological Issues in Mesothelioma: Role of SV40," *Journal of Cell Physiology*, 1999; 180(2):167–72.

6. D. Malkin, "Simian Virus 40 and Non-Hodgkin Lymphoma," *The Lancet*, 2002; 359(9309):812–13.

7. V. Fulginiti, "Killed-Measles-Virus Vaccine," *The Lancet*, 1967; 2:468.

8. S. Kharabsheh et al., "Mass Psychogenic Illness Following Tetanus-Diphtheria Toxoid Vaccination in Jordan," *Bulletin of the World Health Organization*, 2001; 79(8):764–70.

9. These two were bitter rivals, and their appearance together suggested some strong arm-twisting.

10. Named after the brilliant French neurologist Georges Charles Guillain and his associate, Jean-Alexander Barre. Guillain was professor of neurology at the world-famous Hospital de la Salpetriere in Paris.

Chapter 4

1. Congenital disease caused by German measles in pregnancy.

2. "Vaccination: The Issue of Our Times," *Mothering Magazine*, 1997.

Chapter 5

1. Peter Razzel, *Edward Jenner's Cowpox Vaccine*, 2d ed. (U.K.: Caliban Books, 1980).

2. S. A. Plotkin and W. A. Orenstein, eds., *Vaccines*, 3d ed. (W. B. Saunders, 1999).

3. Some individuals vaccinated fifteen to twenty years ago may still be immune—it is unknown exactly how long vaccine-induced immunity lasts.

4. R. Preston, "The Demon in the Freezer," *New Yorker*, July 12, 1999, pp. 44–61.

5. In 1976, Gerald Ford did the same with the swine flu scare, but he received his injection on television.

6. Strictly speaking, only the state can legislate mandatory vaccination, but in practice, the federal government sets policy.

Chapter 6

1. The great pox was, of course, syphilis.

2. William Heberden was perhaps the best and last of eighteenth-century English classical scholars and physicians. He collaborated with Benjamin Franklin in popularizing smallpox vaccination.

3. Usually guinea pig.

4. Advisory Committee for Immunization Practices, a government agency.

5. T. Lieu et al., "Cost-Effectiveness of a Routine Varicella Vaccination Program," *Journal of the American Medical Association*, 1994; 271:375–81.

6. M. Brisson et al., "Varicella Vaccination," *Journal of Medical Virology*, 70 Suppl, 2003; 1:S31–7.

7. Studies show that antibody levels last a long time after immunization, but this is probably because of repeated exposure to natural virus.

8. M. Brisson et al., "Exposure To Varicella Boosts Immunity To Herpes Zoster," *Vaccine*, 2002; 20:2500–2507.

9. The Vaccine is valuable when applied to persons at high risk of severe chicken pox as well as to health care workers.

Chapter 7

1. Ironically, Aretaeus was forgotten after his death until he was rediscovered almost a thousand years later.

2. This dilemma is powerfully dramatized in William Carlos Williams' 1933 "The Use of Force," in which a physician's need to examine his pretty child patient causes him to overcome her resistance by brute force, which may have compromised his professional integrity.

3. Disease or other abnormality of the nerves.

4. For a while the antitoxin was also used as a preventive in case of known exposure to diphtheria, but it never became established in that role.

5. In addition, he added the "von" to his name. In 1968 a newly discovered bacterium, Kitasatoa purperea, was named after Kitasato.

6. The thimerosal issue is discussed elsewhere.

Chapter 8

1. Curiously, these antibodies do not protect the infant from becoming infected.

2. P. Kendrick, "Progress Report on Pertussis Immunization," *American Journal of Public Health*, 1936; 26:8–12.

3. W. Sako, "Studies on Pertussis Immunization," *Journal of Pediatrics*, 1947; 30:29–40.

4. Medical Research Council, "Vaccination against Whooping Cough," *British Medical Journal*, 1959; 1:994–1000.

5. Physicians who looked harder found more cases, making the vaccine appear less effective.

6. C. D. C. Christie, "The 1993 Cincinnati Epidemic of Pertussis," *New England Journal of Medicine*, 1994; 331:16–21.

7. K. M. Edwards et al., "Pertussis Vaccine," in Stanley Plotkin and Walter Orenstein, *Vaccines* (W. B. Saunders, 1999), pp. 406–7.

8. In the absence of immunization, epidemics appear at three-to-five-year intervals. Following an epidemic, almost the whole population is immune. It takes several years before there are enough susceptible children and/or adults to sustain an epidemic.

Chapter 9

1. A close relative of Clostridium tetani produces the foul-smelling gas gangrene. It is usually fatal, but some cases have improved after treatment in high-pressure oxygen chambers.

2. Now a naturalist's paradise.

3. If this proves to be true, the child will in effect be getting its first "shot" before birth!

4. Ellen Bolte, *Autism and Clostridium Tetani, Medical Hypotheses*, 1998; vol. 51: 133–44.

Chapter 11

1. *London Medical Journal*, 1790; 11:190–211.

Chapter 12

1. Robert Kim-Farley, "Rubella," in Kenneth Kiple, *Cambridge World History of Human Disease* (Cambridge University Press, 1993).

Chapter 13

1. The stele can be seen in Copenhagen, Denmark at Ny Carlsberg Glyptotek.

2. Dr. George Draper, who was a great student of polio and personal physician to FDR, unfortunately described the double hump phenomenon as

the dromedary hump, although that camel has but one hump. His fame, sadly, rests more on this error than on his solid achievements in polio research.

3. In the prevaccine era, artificial respiration was accomplished by the "iron lung," an airtight chamber encompassing the whole body except the head and neck. The pressure in the chamber was continuously cycled between positive and negative, thus forcing air into and out of the lungs.

4. Yale University Press, 1995.

5. But FDR was infected in 1921.

6. The electron microscope, invented in 1937, made viruses visible.

7. At its peak, this kind of research was consuming monkeys by the tens of thousands.

8. The March of Dimes was probably the best fund-raising organization of all time.

9. In practice at least two doses are given.

Chapter 14

1. For a modern version of this belief, see Velikovsky's *Worlds in Collision*.

2. It was called the Spanish flu because Spain was a noncombatant during the Great War and, unlike the other European countries, did not try to censor the extent of the epidemic.

3. Kenneth Kiple, ed., *The Cambridge World History of Human Disease* (Cambridge University Press, 1993), p. 808.

4. Ibid.

5. Ten times the number of American combat deaths in the Great War.

6. This was the case in the 1967 swine flu fiasco. The virus appeared to resemble so closely the flu virus of the 1918 disaster.

7. If nonflu respiratory infections are counted as flu cases, the vaccine will appear to be less effective.

8. J. M. Watson et al., "Does influenza immunisation cause exacerbations of chronic airflow obstruction or asthma?" *Thorax*, 1997; 57:190–194.

Chapter 15

1. It was during this period that French scientist Albert Leon Charles Calmette, famous for his development of the TB vaccine, was interned by the Germans. He might have been executed but for the intervention of Pfeiffer, who held the rank of general in the German army.

2. But in pigs and ducks, Hemophilus influenzae seems to work in conjunction with the flu virus.

3. The cartilage flap that keeps food from "going the wrong way" down the windpipe.

Chapter 16

1. Including those who have sickle cell anemia; absence of a spleen; alcoholism, chronic liver, kidney, or heart disease; HIV infection.

2. My guess is that these estimates are "guesstimates."

3. There are strains without capsules; these usually do not cause illness.

4. Usually a fragment of a powerful toxin such as tetanus, diphtheria, or meningococcal antigen.

Chapter 17

1. Cirrhosis and liver cancer occur in the absence of HBV.

2. The volunteers were sometimes the investigators themselves.

Chapter 18

1. In the old days when people smoked cigarettes, the loss of taste for them was said to be an early symptom of hepatitis.

Chapter 19

1. Connelly Smith and Jeffrey Starke, "Bacille Calmette-Guérin Vaccine," in Stanley Plotkin and Walter Orenstein, *Vaccines* (W. B. Saunders, 1999).

2. Kenneth Kiple, ed., *Cambridge World History of Human Disease* (Cambridge University Press, 1993).

3. Ibid. The germ theory of the West was not developed until two hundred years later.

4. Hans Castorp stayed seven years.

5. Singing may be even worse.

6. M. tuberculosis has many cousins; some can cause illness. The question here is whether these organisms have caused a positive skin test.

7. "The usual suspects": the uneducated, poor, homeless, despised minorities, refugees, DPs, drug addicts, alcoholics. They are always with us—the depository and reservoir of disease.

Chapter 20

1. The fifth and sixth Egyptian plagues in 1500 B.C. are believed to have been caused by anthrax.

2. Hence *anthrax*, black, like the coal.

3. I will leave it to the specialists to explain how this life cycle evolved.

4. Even Judge Sullivan questioned this sudden efficiency.

Chapter 21

1. Although this chapter deals only with vaccines, many other measures can be taken to avoid travel illness.

Chapter 22

1. St. Louis, West Nile, La Crosse, Eastern Equine, Western Equine, and Venezuelan.
2. And horses.
3. It will never be eradicated because of its huge reservoir of nonhuman hosts.
4. We have seen a spontaneous decrease of numerous diseases. The usual explanation is improved sanitation, antibiotics, etc. I prefer to think that this phenomenon is due to evolutionary changes in the human/host relationship.

Chapter 23

1. There have been, possibly, six or seven survivors.
2. Invented by J. R. Petri, who worked with Robert Koch, Pasteur's archrival.
3. There have been exceptionally rare cases of a rabid dog outliving its victim.

Chapter 24

1. Serial passage through various animals or cell cultures, culture in cold conditions, other manipulations—see previous chapter.
2. There is also a live polio vaccine.
3. In this context, "vector" is the equivalent of "carrier."
4. Recently nasal flu vaccine was licensed, but it has not had great success.
5. Prohibitively in many parts of the world.
6. But let's note that William B. Coley, a surgeon, attempted to produce an anticancer vaccine in 1880. He discovered that a high level of generalized immunity could be achieved by injection of bacterial toxins. The antibody responses to Coley's toxin attacked the cancer cells. He had some remarkable success, but many failures. Side effects were severe and frequent. With the advent of radiation therapy and chemotherapy, Coley's toxin was relegated to the quackery category until its rehabilitation by his daughter's work in immunology. Coley's toxin was discontinued by Parke-Davis in the fifties, but it is still used in some quarters.

Chapter 25

1. Richard Horton, *New York Review of Books*, September 23, 2004.

2. I will use "AIDS" to refer to any stage of HIV infection, and will use "HIV" to refer to the virus.

3. Hooper's book is a tour de force but never proves even the possibility of a polio vaccine causing AIDS. Genetic analyses of the evolution of HIV has further discredited Hooper's hypothesis. Edward Hooper, *The River: A Journey to the Source of HIV and AIDS*, Penguin Press, 1999.

4. 10 followed by eight zeros.

5. Some patients who had come to terms with their impending death (and even cashed in their insurance policies) became angry when told they were going to live.

6. Note how the patient has become a subject and the clinician an investigator.

7. "For every human problem, there is a neat, simple solution; and it is always wrong." H. L. Mencken (1880–1956), Mencken's Metalaw.

8. The same is true for counseling subjects on AIDS prevention. Some studies have the counseling being done by individuals not associated with the study.

9. Amanda Silverio, "HIV Research in Africa: A Series of Paradoxes," *Stanford Journal of International Relations* (at www.stanford.edu/group/sjir/ 3.2.05__silverio.html).

Appendix B

1. Allergy, immune deficiency, contact with immune-deficient persons, asthma, eczema.

2. A nice Catch-22: You can't go to school without the shots, but it's against the law not to attend school. Home schooling does not avoid the issue; the state requires that the shots be given anyway.

3. Some states do not require children to receive whooping cough vaccine, others do not require mumps vaccine, but both of these are available only in combination with other, required vaccines.

4. The director, Division of Vaccine Injury Compensation, Bureau of Health Professions, Health Resources and Services Administration; the deputy director for Scientific Activities, Office of the Assistant Secretary of Defense for Health Affairs, Department of Defense; the undersecretary for Health, Department of Veterans Affairs; the director, Center for Biologics Evaluation and Research, Food and Drug Administration; the director, Center for Medicaid and State Operations, Health Care Financing Administration; the director, Division of Microbiology and Infectious Diseases, National Institute of Allergy

and Infectious Diseases, National Institutes of Health; the director, Indian Health Service, Department of Health and Human Services; and the director, National Vaccine Program Office, Centers for Disease Control and Prevention.

5. See the section on swine flu vaccine and the Ford/Reagan contest.
6. Clever fellows.
7. Or even the doctors.

Appendix C

1. All treatments sometimes have adverse effects.
2. Aspirin, zinc, and antibiotics "cure" a cold in seven days.
3. Such as selecting the healthier looking (or sicker) individuals.
4. This has been a special problem in AIDS research.

Index

ABOUT THE AUTHOR

KURT LINK, M.D., is Assistant Professor of Medicine at Virginia Commonwealth University. He has been practicing internal medicine for more than 35 years. Dr. Link was educated at the Bronx High School of Science, City College of New York and Albert Einstein College of Medicine of Yeshiva University.